REVIEWS

"With a primary care physician's empathy, skill, and experience, Dr. Hanna explains the dire consequences of the American healthcare non-system. And like good primary care, *Dying of Health Care* does not abandon the reader after delivering this grave diagnosis. Dr. Hanna recommends practical solutions to put us on the path back to better individual health and national well-being. Americans simply cannot afford to ignore the ideas so clearly presented in this book."

> —John Abramson, M.D., M.Sc. Lecturer in the Department of Health Care Policy at Harvard Medical School and author of *Overdosed America: The Broken Promise of American Medicine*

"Many Americans believe our health care system is broken, but can't describe how or why. In his new book *Dying of Health Care*, Dr. N.F. Hanna offers an intriguing taxonomy of the many interwoven factors that add up to a badly broken system, and how to fix it from the perspective of an experienced clinician.

This book is a must-read for anybody who has been, is, or will be a patient. That's just about all of us."

> —Philip Caper, M.D. Internist, past Chairman of the National Council on Health Planning and Development, and Founding Member of the National Academy of Social Insurance

---

"Dr. N.F. Hanna's *Dying of Health Care* is a welcome addition to the American medical care literature. An experienced primary care physician, Hanna brings that practical understanding to the most basic questions about the costs, quality, and access to care of our expensive, underinsured, and exceedingly complex medical arrangements."

> —Ted Marmor, Ph.D. Professor Emeritus of Public Policy at Yale University and author of *The Politics of Medicare*, among other books

"Dr. Hanna's *Dying of Health Care* provides a lucid and accessible analysis of the many ways that American medical practices, and the financial institutions profiting from the business of medicine, make us less healthy than we deserve to be, while making medicine far more dangerous than it should be. This book deserves a wide reading."

> —Larry R. Churchill, Ph.D. Anne Geddes Stahlman Professor of Medical Ethics at Vanderbilt University

"Hanna has provided a thoughtful, engaging analysis of why there is so much waste in the U.S. health care system, and he exposes the financial and human costs of unnecessary care. As a solution, he eloquently argues for the creation of a single-payer system. Even those who disagree with the idea of a single-payer system will benefit from this insightful and important critique."

> —Kenneth Ludmerer, M.D. Professor of Medicine and the History of Medicine at Washington University in St. Louis, past President of the American Association for the History of Medicine, and member of the American Academy of Arts and Sciences

Dying of Health Care

How the System Harms Americans
Physically and Financially,
and How to Change It

N.F. Hanna, M.D.

Dying of Health Care:
*How the System Harms Americans Physically and Financially,
and How to Change It*

First Edition

Copyright © 2016 N.F. Hanna, M.D. All rights reserved.

ISBN-13: 978-1542770095

ISBN-10: 1542770092

DEDICATION

To my former colleagues at Ormskirk General Hospital in Lancashire, England. It was with them that I learned, taught, conferred, and developed an understanding of the subjectivity of medical decision-making, as well as the enormity of the impact that these decisions have on both the quantity and health-related quality of patients' lives.

CONTENTS

Introduction — 1

Section I. Setting the Stage

Chapter One
The Paradox of Paying More to Get Less — 7

Chapter Two
The Intertwining of Physical, Emotional, and Financial Well-Being — 15

Chapter Three
Understanding Medical Decision-Making — 25

Section II. The Diagnosis: Paying More

Section II, Part A. Costs Caused Primarily by the Medical Profession

Chapter Four
Excessive Testing — 39

Chapter Five
Doctors Overprescribing — 49

Chapter Six
Bypassing the Primary Care Physician:
Direct-to-Specialist Referrals and Consultations — 55

Chapter Seven
Doctors Not Assessing the Costs to the System — 61

Section II, Part B. Costs Caused by Other Factors

Chapter Eight
The Health Insurance and Medical Billing Industries:
The Two Middlemen   67

Chapter Nine
Overpriced Pharmaceuticals and Medical Devices:
Manufacturer Price Gouging and Deceptive Practices   73

Chapter Ten
A Fragmented Hospital System with High Overhead Costs   79

Chapter Eleven
Ever-Increasing Administrative Costs for Medical Practices   83

Chapter Twelve
Direct-to-Consumer Marketing by Pharmaceutical Companies   89

Section III. The Diagnosis: Getting Less

Chapter Thirteen
Iatrogenic Diseases: The Third Most Common
Cause of Death in the United States   95

Chapter Fourteen
Dissecting Iatrogenic Diseases   103

Section IV. Preparing for the Prescription

Chapter Fifteen
From Macroeconomics to Health Care Economics:
Why Our Path is Unsustainable   113

Chapter Sixteen
Getting Immunized Against Journalistic Sensationalism
and Political Demagoguery   123

Section V. Prescribing the Treatment

Chapter Seventeen
Create a Single-Payer with Authority ... 129

Chapter Eighteen
Standardize Medical Decision-Making ... 137

Chapter Nineteen
Improve Training of Primary Care Physicians
to Be the Anchors of Health Care ... 143

Chapter Twenty
Implement Medical Malpractice Reform ... 147

Chapter Twenty-One
A Pilot Program:
Implement Self-Contained Community Health Centers ... 149

Section VI. A Call to Action

Chapter Twenty-Two
From Teddy Roosevelt to Barack Obama and Beyond:
The Quest for Universal, Affordable Health Care Continues ... 155

Chapter Twenty-Three
No Time to Wait ... 165

Chapter Twenty-Four
Fulfilling a Century-Long Dream: Rising Above Politics
to Achieve Universal, Affordable Health Care ... 169

Endnotes ... 173

About the Author ... 191

ACKNOWLEDGMENTS

I would like to share my appreciation for the tireless efforts of my daughter Amorette and son Andrew in helping me complete this book. Without them, this would not have been possible!

INTRODUCTION

Despite our many differences, all of us have at least one thing in common: health care is central to our lives. Good health is the single most influential factor in the well-being of any person, regardless of socio-economic class, ethnicity, age, gender, background, or where in the world you live. Sadly, the American health care system, in my own view and in the view of so many others, is ailing and needs treatment. Every attempt to diagnose and treat the problem in the past has been either shortsighted or too focused on a small portion of the problem. These attempts have been piecemeal, band-aid approaches; they have not been comprehensive, nor have they fully examined the major role the medical profession plays as part of the problems as well as the potential solutions. If the flaws in our country's health care system are not addressed and treated promptly, they will threaten both the physical and financial well-being of our families and our nation as a whole. Yet, the conversation sometimes seems too complex and convoluted to discuss real, comprehensive, and durable solutions. I hope that this book helps to change that.

    Before I go on, a bit of background on myself: I am a primary care physician practicing in Jacksonville, Florida. I was born and raised in Egypt and graduated from medical school in the capital city of Cairo. I have been practicing medicine in the United States for almost 30 years as a solo practitioner, preceded by about six years of practicing in the United Kingdom. Having witnessed two nearly diametrically opposed systems of health care delivery in these countries (an almost entirely public system in the U.K. and a mostly private system in the U.S.), I have developed what I believe is a unique perspective on the pitfalls and benefits of each. Experiencing two different systems that are often compared to one another, and experiencing them specifically as a primary care physician in the center of the health care delivery system, is a luxury not many doctors get a chance to have.

Because I have practiced for so many years as a primary care physician in one place, I have seen many hundreds of patients quite regularly for almost three decades. Needless to say, I have developed strong bonds with them. We as primary care physicians enjoy a unique relationship with our patients because we are the first and continuous point of contact for all of their health care needs. As a result of this special bond, we get to know our patients very well and are equipped to treat not just the disease, but the patient as well. I have celebrated my patients' joys and triumphs, but also mourned with them in their deepest tragedies and sorrows. I have shared and continue to share in their trials and tribulations in life – and not merely as their doctor. I have at times assumed the role of their friend, their confidant, their advocate, and even their family member; they sometimes confide in me things they do not even share with their own families or members of their clergy. Ultimately, I have gotten to know their inner selves very well, from their insecurities to their greatest joys. Indeed, these close relationships make it so that I am not just a casual observer of the health care problems we are facing as a nation.

It is from these experiences that I have developed the ideas in this book. I view the patients I see and care for as a microcosm of the larger universe of Americans living within our health care system. So, fixing these problems means the world to me because it means the world to my patients.

An Overview of What is to Come
With this in mind, my intention is to take a critical look at the U.S. health care system from the perspective of a physician with deep experience within it. As is taught in medical school, it all starts with diagnosing the problem. We will diagnose the challenges facing our health care system and the root causes contributing to each. I will

illustrate these issues by sharing examples of patients I have seen, helping to put faces to the problems we explore. We will then prescribe innovative treatments and highlight the groups of people that can step up to solve these problems. Note that some of the analyses and concepts of both the "diagnosis" and the "treatment" discussed in this book are original and have never been discussed or presented in any forum, nor have they appeared in any publication to date. Here is how we will proceed:

The Diagnosis: If you misdiagnose, the treatment will be irrelevant. A correct diagnosis is pivotal. So, before the diagnosis, we must set the stage properly. We will start by understanding the magnitude of the problems facing our health care system by considering a key paradox: Americans pay considerably more for health care than our counterparts in other developed nations, and yet we are falling short in nearly all metrics of health, including life expectancy. Put simply, we are paying more for health care and getting less... literally less of life, both in terms of quantity and health-related quality. We will then explore how, in this current system, physical ailment leads to financial and emotional ailment, dramatically damaging the overall well-being of people. Finally, I will take you into the mind of a doctor, where medical decisions are made. The highly subjective nature of medical decision-making has enormous bearing on both the outcome of the treatment and its costs. All of this background will make for strong preparation for our diagnosis.

The diagnosis itself follows. We will explore the root causes of the paradox: first why we are paying more and then why we are getting less. Within the "Paying More" portion, we will explore the costs caused primarily by the medical profession (as a doctor, I specifically hope to shed some light on the role of our profession in contributing to both aspects of the paradox, as well as its potential in contributing to the solutions) and costs not caused by the medical profession (for these, doctors and patients alike are victims of other players in the system). In the "Getting Less" section, we will explore something I will refer to as the "dual death" of the American patient – both a physical death and a financial death. The physical death comes in the cases in which doctors' medical or surgical interventions actually cause death. These cases, as we will see, are called "iatrogenic diseases," or doctor-made diseases, and they are estimated to be the third most common cause of death in the U.S. The financial death comes in the form of personal financial burdens and ultimately bankruptcy (which is akin to the death of a person as a financial entity). Medical expenses are by far the number one cause of this "financial death" in the United States. In all of this, the economic implications for our government and our corporations are enormous, and the current state of affairs is simply unsustainable.

The Treatment: This all seems quite daunting, but there is most certainly hope. In medicine, a doctor often must prepare the patient for the treatment, particularly if it will be a tough one to hear – even if it is the only way to the cure. In the same way, the "Preparing for the Prescription" section will consider the crucial-to-understand economics of health care and the need to avoid being caught in the journalistic sensationalism and political demagoguery that so often clouds our ability to honestly evaluate ideas. When it is finally time for "Prescribing the Treatment," we will then consider five main ideas – some novel and others that have been discussed before – that can truly work to fix our health care system. Thankfully, as we will see, so many of the solutions meant to help better treat patients will also reduce health care costs and make quality care more affordable at the same time. It is a most beautiful case of the proverbial "killing two birds with one stone."

Together, we must decide to push aside entrenched ideological arguments that simply detract from what the real topic should be: making sure every American has quality and affordable health care. Debates and discussions on health care reform in the United States are perhaps reaching a crescendo after more than one hundred years of nearly continuous debate. We have a fantastic opportunity today as citizens to take action and ensure that patients are put first.

I sincerely hope that this book provides insight, awareness, and ideas that will transform our health care system into one that provides Americans with quality, universal, affordable health care that is economically sustainable for us as well as future generations.

Let us begin.

SECTION I.
SETTING THE STAGE

CHAPTER ONE
THE PARADOX OF PAYING MORE TO GET LESS

The Problem with Our Health Care System... in a Nutshell
To begin to understand the problem with the American health care system, just two simple facts need to be presented:

1. We pay far more for health care than any other Western industrial nation.

2. Yet, we are considerably behind in most metrics of health care quality.

Throughout this book, we will dive into the specific contributors that make these two facts a reality. We will draw on my experiences as a physician, consider real life examples of my own patients, and explore potential innovative solutions. For now, however, we will lay the groundwork and see, on a larger scale, just how enormous and impossible to ignore the problem currently is.

Paying More
To illustrate the first point – that we are paying more – let us take a look at some statistics.

When compared to the other 33 developed nations in the Organization for Economic Cooperation and Development (OECD), the United States spends considerably more on health care. Based on the OECD Health Statistics 2014 report, the U.S. had the highest total per person health expenditure: $8,745 per person in 2012. The nation with the second highest total health expenditure per person was Norway, coming in well behind the U.S. at $6,140 per person.[1] The United States spends more than two times what is spent on health care per person in most developed countries in the world, including France, Sweden, and the U.K.,[2] where I myself practiced medicine for six years before coming to America. When you total it all up, the Center for Medicare and Medicaid Services (CMS) found that the U.S. spent an estimated $2.9 trillion in 2013 on health care.[3] Just to make sure we at least attempt to absorb this enormous figure, that is $2,900,000,000,000. The same analysis estimated health care spending in the U.S. would reach over $3.2 trillion in 2015, which is $10,000 *per person*. What is worse is that, as shown in a Thomson Reuters study in 2009, experts estimated that up to one-third of our spending at the time – between $505 billion and $850 billion – went towards care that was inefficient, wasteful, or redundant.[4]

One may point out that the United States is the richest nation on the list and *should* be spending more on health care. Even when factoring in the wealth of a country, however, we see in Figure 1.1 below that the U.S. (shown at the far left of the graph) dramatically outspends any other nation in the world.[5]

Figure 1.1
Health Expenditure, Public and Private,
as a Share of GDP in OECD Countries, 2012 or Latest Year

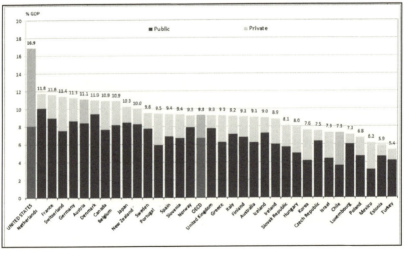

Source: OECD Health Statistics 2014

When looking at total health expenditure in terms of percentage of gross domestic product (GDP) as opposed to per person, we still see the same trend. As seen in the graph on the previous page, American health care costs gobbled up 16.9 percent of our national GDP in 2012. Again, this high value far overshadows all other nations in the OECD. It is nearly two times the OECD average (9.3 percent) and far above the second highest nation, the Netherlands, with 11.8 percent of Dutch GDP going to health care.[6] Spending on nearly every component of health care is higher in the U.S. than it is in these other countries.

Getting Less

It would seem reasonable that the U.S. spends far more on health care than any other nation in the world, so long as our health results are the best in the world as well. Unfortunately, this is very far from the truth.

To evaluate this, there are several studies that consider a variety of health metrics and rank the health care systems of nations around the world. The common conclusion across all of them: the U.S. is not delivering the quality that the price tag would suggest. And, truthfully, it is not even close.

A 2014 study by the Commonwealth Fund ranked the health care systems of 11 developed nations and found that the U.S. ranked *last* overall, while the U.K. ranked first. This study considered factors such as quality of care, access to doctors, and equity throughout the country.[7] As just one other example, take the World Health Organization (WHO) report from 2000, when it conducted the first-ever full analysis of the world's health care systems. Using five performance indicators to evaluate health systems in 191 countries, it found that the U.S. ranked just 37th in overall health system performance.[8]

To get into every category in which the American system performs poorly would take quite a while, so let us only consider a couple of examples. For one, the 2014 OECD report cites the fact that the U.S. had only 3.1 hospital beds per 1,000 people in 2010, ranking us 25th out of the 34 OECD nations.[9] For comparison,

Japan, the global leader, had 13.4 beds and Germany had 8.3 beds per 1,000 people in 2012.[10] The U.S. also has fewer doctors per person than most developed countries. We had 2.5 practicing physicians per 1,000 people in 2011, ranking us 28th out of the 34 OECD nations.[11]

In my opinion, life expectancy is the best metric to consider in evaluating a health care system because it is the cumulative effect of all aspects of health. It cannot be explained away, especially when it is considered in a comparison of similar countries like those within the OECD. I believe this metric paints the most accurate picture of health care, and it does not reflect positively on the American system.

Like the rest of the world, the U.S. has had recent increases in terms of life expectancy. However, we once again pale in comparison on the global level. American life expectancy increased by almost nine years between 1960 and 2010, however this is below the OECD average increase of 11 years. According to the OECD Health Statistics from 2014, the U.S. ranks 27th out of the 34 OECD countries in terms of life expectancy at birth (recall that in the same report, the U.S. ranked 1st among the OECD countries in terms of total health expenditure).[12] The 2014 World Health Organization annual report shows that, per 2012 statistics, the average American woman lives until the age of 81, while women in Japan live six years longer with a life expectancy of 87. The disparities exist for men as well. American male life expectancy is 76 years, while it is 80 years in Japan and even higher in seven other countries.[13] The U.S. ranks 42nd in the world in terms of life expectancy at birth according to the Central Intelligence Agency's (CIA) World Factbook, and it is does not crack the upper echelon of the rankings for either gender.[14] The World Economic Forum (WEF), in its Global Competitiveness Report of 2014-2015, found similar results, as it has the U.S. ranked 34th out of 144 countries in terms of life expectancy at birth.[15]

We can also consider other metrics, like infant mortality rate. This is the number of deaths of children less than one year old per 1,000 live births. It is a good indicator of a country's health system because it speaks to many different areas like maternal care and access to care. According to the CIA's 2013 World Factbook, the infant mortality rate in the U.S. is 6.17 (so 6.17 deaths per 1,000 live births), which ranks 56th of the 224 countries listed (in other words, 55 countries had lower infant mortality rates than the U.S.).[16] A 2014 report by the Center for Disease Control and Prevention (CDC) showed that the U.S. infant mortality rate ranked last in a comparison of 26 developed countries (see Figure 1.2 below).[17] For perspective, the U.S. rate is more than 2.5 times that of Japan and Finland. The World Economic Forum in 2014 found that the U.S. ranks lowly in this area as well, standing at 39th in the world.[18]

Figure 1.2
Infant Mortality Rates in Selected OECD Countries, 2010

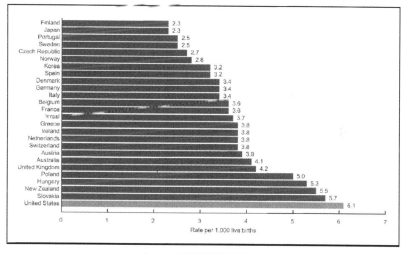

Sources: CDC/NCHS, OECD

While the U.S. health care system does excel in some areas, perhaps most notably the area of cancer treatment, one thing is unquestionably clear through all the numbers, statistics, and comparisons: *the performance is significantly behind where it should be given the amount of money we are paying.* The situation is summed up well in this quote from a study published in *The Journal of the American Medical Association* (JAMA) in 2013:

"The United States spends the most per capita on health care across all countries, lacks universal health coverage, and lags behind other high-income countries for life expectancy and many other health outcome measures. High costs with mediocre population health outcomes at the national level are compounded by marked disparities across communities, socioeconomic groups, and race and ethnicity groups."[19]

Shopping for a Life… Literally
No consumer, no matter what degree of prudence he or she may have, would accept paying more for goods or services to get less when compared to others. In a way, as consumers of health care, we are quite literally shopping for life. To put together our analysis of paying more and getting less, consider this comparison: in 2012, the U.S. spent $8,745 per capita in total health expenditures, with a total population life expectancy at birth of 78.8 years. Meanwhile in Spain, during the same year, the total health expenditures came to $2,928 per capita, and life expectancy was 82.5 years.[20] Indeed, it is when you combine our previous look at how much more we are paying as Americans with this consideration of how much less we are getting in terms of life expectancy that things get *really* shocking. Figure 1.3 on the following page plots the life expectancy of several countries against per-person health care spending in 2013. In reading the chart, the most efficient and effective systems fall in the upper left area. From our conversation thus far, you would expect the U.S. to be an outlier in that its system is so expensive and not as effective. But saying it is an outlier is a major understatement. Note particularly how far the U.S.'s life expectancy mark falls below the trend curve, which is where you would expect it to fall based on its amount of spending.[21] Sadly, as Americans, we are simply paying more and getting less than people in many other countries.

Figure 1.3
Life Expectancy at Birth and Health Spending Per Capita in OECD Countries, 2011 or Latest Year

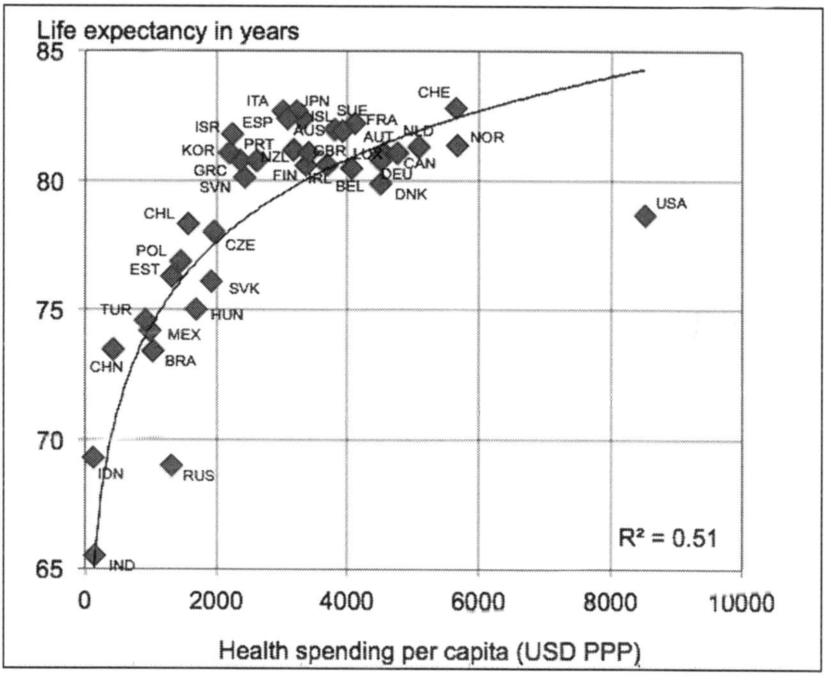

[Scatter plot: Life expectancy in years (y-axis, 65–85) vs. Health spending per capita (USD PPP) (x-axis, 0–10000). Countries plotted include ITA, JPN, ISL, SWE, FRA, CHE, ISR, ESP, AUS, AUT, NLD, KOR, PRT, NZL, GBR, LUX, NOR, GRC, FIN, IRL, CAN, SVN, BEL, DEU, DNK, USA, CHL, POL, EST, CZE, SVK, TUR, HUN, MEX, BRA, CHN, IDN, RUS, IND. $R^2 = 0.51$.]

Source: OECD Health Statistics 2013

Moving Forward

Of course, we must move forward and analyze the problems more deeply so that we can offer remedies. With this broad understanding of the challenge that is facing the American health care system and, consequently, the American people, we can begin to look more carefully at the components of the problem. Most importantly, we can propose specific and innovative solutions that can help solve this conundrum of paying more while getting less; these are solutions that go far beyond ideologically driven debates and seek to make changes that our country desperately and urgently needs.

CHAPTER TWO
THE INTERTWINING OF PHYSICAL, EMOTIONAL, AND FINANCIAL WELL-BEING

The role of a primary care physician (PCP) is a truly unique one in the medical profession. We often assume different roles that extend far beyond being merely a family physician. As mentioned in the Introduction, we develop bonds over time that go much further than just treating illnesses; we are often treating the patients themselves. This includes aspects of their psychosocial lives, which have a critical bearing on their physical health.

From this up close and personal standpoint, I have seen over the years that the physical, emotional, and financial health of a patient are closely tied together. All three aspects of a person's health are crucially and inseparably intertwined. They go hand-in-hand almost all the time; any one of the three can adversely, or positively, affect the other two.

Too many times I have seen serious, unexpected illnesses – in addition to physically threatening their health – totally destroy the savings that my patients have built up over the course of their lifetimes. Of course, when these patients find themselves without the means to support their families or sometimes to even survive, there is an unbearable psychological impact and that, in turn, affects their physical health. It is a bitterly vicious cycle that continues to spiral downward.

If a patient is not insured, one serious illness can lead to huge medical bills and financial ruin. A serious illness that leaves a patient physically disabled, too, can take away his or her earning power. Needless to say, this leads to emotional upheaval in both circumstances. Even if a patient is insured, catastrophic illness can have an enormous financial and thus emotional consequence, even in the absence of disability.

Medical Bills: The Number One Cause of Bankruptcies
The facts suggest that what I have described is an all-too-common problem. Many sources cite medical reasons as the number one cause of personal bankruptcies across the United States, an even more common cause than credit card bills or unpaid mortgages. NerdWallet Health analyzed data from the U.S. Census, the Center for Disease Control, the federal court system, and the Commonwealth Fund in order to better understand how common it is for Americans to struggle with medical bills. The study revealed that, in 2013, three in five bankruptcies were due to medical bills.[1] A study conducted by Harvard University indicated that 62.1 percent of all bankruptcies in 2007, using a conservative definition, were medical bankruptcies. The study showed that for 92 percent of the medically bankrupt, high medical bills directly contributed to their bankruptcy. Using identical definitions and controlling for demographic factors, the same study found that the odds a bankruptcy had a medical cause in 2007 were 2.38 times higher than in 2001,[2] indicating a troubling trend. Of course, filing for bankruptcy goes far beyond financial pain. There is also the immense emotional burden of starting over and the social pressure – even shame – which can be involved.

Beyond Bankruptcy: Iatrogenic Poverty
Not everyone who struggles will choose to go as far as declaring bankruptcy, but this does not mean health care costs are not a distressing burden in these people's lives. According to 2012 National Health Interview Survey (NHIS) data, 20 percent of non-elderly adults reported struggling with medical bills in the previous year. When the definition was broadened to include those who have had problems affording medical bills over a longer period of time, and those unable to pay some medical bills at all, nearly one

in three (32 percent) reported having medical bill problems.[3]

Some have labeled the phenomenon in which medical costs drive an individual or family into dire financial straits as "iatrogenic poverty." Iatrogenic diseases, as we will see later on, are doctor-made diseases; they are diseases that are caused by medical intervention. Accordingly, iatrogenic poverty is doctor-made poverty. It is poverty that is a direct result of medical treatment, specifically its costs. The cost of treatment, when added to the many other costs of the illness itself (foregone wages, decreased productivity, and more), incurs devastating consequences that push the individual into financial shock, leading to financial risk-taking that often drives the person into poverty.[4] The concept of iatrogenic poverty is just another illustration of the interweaving of physical, financial, and emotional well-being. In truth, we should not have to live in insecurity, always vulnerable to iatrogenic poverty. But so many do, and certainly not just the uninsured.

Insurance Is Not Enough
Yes, even those with insurance struggle mightily. The aforementioned Harvard study revealed that over three quarters (78 percent) of medical debtors were insured at the onset of illness.[5] Indeed, a case study by the Henry J. Kaiser Family Foundation (KFF) concluded that while the chances of falling into medical debt are greater for people without insurance, the majority of people who experience difficulty paying medical bills are people with health insurance. KFF's study echoed the fact that the vast majority of those affected by medical debt – it estimated 70 percent – are actually insured (see Figure 2.1 on the following page).[6]

I often see patients who are considered "underinsured;" they have insurance plans with very high deductibles (the amount of money a person pays before the insurance kicks in) in order to have more affordable premiums (the amount of money a person pays on a regular basis). These patients sometimes wait extraordinarily long periods of time before seeking medical help in order to avoid paying that high deductible. Sometimes, if the symptoms occur in the second half of the year, these patients are tempted to wait to see a doctor in order to have their deductible paid early in the new year. As a consequence of these behaviors, so many underinsured patients wait until their medical problems have gotten much more severe and less easily treatable. They are actually paying with their own lives! Again, these medical struggles deal a heavy physical, emotional, and financial blow.

Figure 2.1
Characteristics of People
with Difficulty Paying Medical Bills

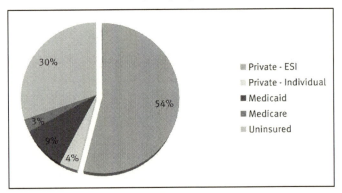

Source: The Henry J. Kaiser Family Foundation

Beyond the examples of my own patients that we will explore later, we can look at the nearly two dozen case studies of people struggling with medical debt explored by Kaiser in partnership with ClearPoint Credit Counseling Services. The case studies included a wide-ranging array of Americans including a 59 year-old trucker named Ben, a 36 year-old financial adviser named Richard, a 58 year-old self-employed accountant named Louise, a 64 year-old retiree named Jeanne, and a 22 year-old restaurant worker named Safiya. In exploring the lives and experiences of such a diverse group of individuals with diverse incomes, family structures, and more, Kaiser found some common themes that are quite telling.

For one, the study found that medical debt can affect just about anyone. The people in the case studies had incomes ranging from under $10,000 to over $100,000 a year. They ranged in age from 22 to 64 in locations all across the country. All but three were insured. For most, this was the first time they struggled with medical debt. Illnesses, accidents, or pregnancies often led to these instances of debt. The message here – one that many of us know all too well – is that there are so many occurrences and difficulties in life that cannot be planned, and they often lead to medical debt.

The study also found that once medical debt starts, it can be hard to stop. Further, it can trigger a cascade of other severe consequences, including bankruptcy, damaged credit ratings, barriers to care, shame, lost homes to foreclosure, depleted retirement or college savings, and countless other challenges. The debt is hard to stop because of new debts – like credit card financing charges – arising from the mechanisms used to pay the original medical debt. Fifteen of the interviewed used credit cards to pay at least some of their outstanding medical bills, which led to financing charges that in turn increased debt.[7]

We sometimes forget in discussions like this that the medical bill was caused by something in the first place – a health issue. The health issue that triggered the downward spiral likely does not go away overnight either. In the vast majority of Kaiser's case studies, the medical problem led to inability to work or reduced hours, which in turn exacerbated the person's financial situation.

I am quite sure that many of you reading right now can relate to this pain – the physical pain that starts the problem, the financial pain of the bills, and the psychological and emotional pain of feeling squeezed for money and having to choose between your family's health and your ability to stay financially afloat. It is an impossible decision to make. The unexpected problems of life are hard enough as it is, but having to worry about medical debt, even with insurance, is simply unfair.

Real Life Encounters
For me, having practiced in the same location and having seen hundreds of the same patients for nearly three decades, this is way beyond numbers and hypotheticals. It is personal.

I could perhaps fill an entire book with heartbreaking stories that I have heard from patients over the years related to the costs of health care and their inability to access quality care. I will bring some of these up throughout this book, using pseudonyms to keep the patients' real identities completely private. For now, it might be helpful to share a few accounts to illustrate just a sliver of the pain that Americans across the country deal with every day. Whether these stories resonate with us because of personal experience or not, it is critical that we as a compassionate society know what is happening and discuss it more thoroughly.

The following are examples of patients I have had over the years, specifically those whose psychosocial lives were influenced by their need to be financially secure in the face of unexpected catastrophic illness. I share these examples to drive home the connection between emotional, financial, and physical health.

1. *I once had a patient – let us call her Anne – whose husband of 30 years passed away. At age 62, Anne subsequently married another man. I found out from her later that this man used to physically assault and beat her. Anne expressed to me that she certainly did not love the man. Of course, I asked her, 'Why did you marry him?'*

   Anne's response: 'Because he had great health insurance.' So, Anne felt that she had to suffer through the physical and emotional ramifications of her marriage simply for the security of having health insurance (which, as we have seen, does not even provide the level of security it should). At 64 and a half, Anne filed for divorce, because she would soon be eligible for Medicare (the national health insurance program for citizens 65 years of age and older). Quality, affordable health care was so precious and difficult to attain for Anne that it became a reason to marry an abusive man with whom she did not want to be.

2. *Another patient of mine was at the time of this story an associate professor at a university. This patient had carefully and responsibly saved for retirement, and he was excited to see that he had enough*

savings to retire before the age of 60. However, he was held back because getting an individual health insurance policy on his own, as opposed to a group policy, was too difficult and expensive due to his relatively poor health (which was still not enough to qualify him for Social Security disability benefits). So he had to continue working until age 65, at which time he would qualify for Medicare. His hard work and planning for so many years did not come to fruition.

3. *A 75 year-old man – let us call him Howard – had multiple diseases that left him unable to take care of himself. Howard's wife had died a few years earlier. Because the cost of a nursing home was far higher than her own salary, Howard's daughter had to give up her job to be a full-time caretaker for her father. Howard, like 90 percent of elderly Americans, did not have private long-term care insurance.[8] In order for Howard to qualify for Medicaid (the national health care program for citizens with low income and limited resources) to cover nursing home costs, the family would have been forced to give all of its assets to the state. After the emotionally difficult event of his wife dying, Howard's physical and financial needs in turn became a difficult physical, financial, and emotional burden for his daughter to bear.*

4. *A 64 year-old professional postponed surgery for a severe carotid artery stenosis (narrowing of one of the arteries supplying blood to the brain). This meant taking the risk of having a stroke while waiting for a year. Why would he take such a risk? It would be a year before he would become eligible for Medicare, and he would have had to pay at least ten thousand dollars out-of-pocket as co-insurance (payments of a share of the amount insurance covers after the deductible is met) if he had used his commercial insurance. Under Medicare, on the other hand, he would pay nothing out of pocket and his commercial insurance would be a secondary one.*

5. *A 52 year-old woman who was a smoker had a mild, lingering cough for a few months, which she thought of as "smoker's cough." She did not seek medical help because she had a five thousand dollar deductible that she felt she could not afford to pay. At a later date, she found out*

that the cough was due to lung cancer that by that time had already spread. She died a few months later.

Contrast these cases to the "over-insured" patients we will discuss in Chapter 7 who want to have a lot of tests done, needed or not, because they have no out-of-pocket expenses. Truly, what we have is an inequitable system. The word "inequitable" often leads diehard political ideologues from the far right of the political spectrum to see this as a call for socialism. However, a reminder should be made to these critics that these "underinsured" patients in the last four examples are all citizens in the middle class or higher; the poor are already covered by Medicaid. These are truly issues that affect nearly all of us.

These patient encounters come from years prior, before the Affordable Care Act. So there is no telling how many of these patients, if any, would have fared better under the new legislation. My guess, judging from my own patients' experiences with Obamacare, is that the first patient would have fared better because she would have had assistance in getting insurance, and the second patient would have been partly helped due to the removal of discrimination against pre-existing diseases. However, the other three patients would have likely fared worse because of the increase in insurance premiums. Because of this, a good deal of patients can only afford insurance with a high deductible and co-insurance. Stories like these show the connection between physical, emotional, and financial health. And, stated simply, stories like these are utterly heartbreaking and should not exist in our society. Of course, there is an element of personal responsibility that must be expected, however the system made it difficult for these patients to exercise it. In the six years that I practiced in the U.K., I never once saw a financial problem related to health care. The problems in the example cases – high insurance premiums, high co-insurance, high deductibles – generally do not exist in public health care systems.

There is no reason for these hardships to occur. Money and health care should never collide, from the patients' and health care providers' perspective alike. When physical and financial health collide, emotional health is an inevitable victim. If the health care-related lack of financial security and its adverse impact on emotional well-being were a health care metric, the U.S. would probably score dead last compared to other developed nations.

CHAPTER THREE
UNDERSTANDING MEDICAL DECISION-MAKING

Before looking at the specific problems and potential solutions in this broken health care system, it is crucial that we explore one more thing: the way doctors generally work. The subjectivity inherent in medical decision-making must be front-and-center in considering the issues of quality and cost of health care. Every day, doctors are making decisions about what diagnostic tests to order and ultimately what modality of treatment to recommend. This, in turn, affects both the outcome of the treatment and its costs to the system. These choices contribute to both ends of the paradox of paying more and getting less, sometimes affecting them adversely at the same time. As you will see in the upcoming chapters on iatrogenic (doctor-caused) diseases and death, there are some instances in which patients can be injured or killed because of medical or surgical intervention. And the costs financially are enormous as well.

Most efforts to analyze the root causes of the outlined dichotomy of paying more and getting less have targeted the cost, blaming various players in the health care industry from pharmaceutical companies to insurers to device manufacturers. Interestingly, the medical profession has been almost completely left out of the equation. It is often considered the innocent bystander in all of this. In reality, as you will see, it is a crucial part of the problem as well as an integral part of the necessary solution.

In this chapter, I will strive to take you into the inner workings of a doctor's mind to help those who are not medically-trained understand a bit more about what is behind a physician's decision-making processes, why these decisions differ from one doctor to another, and how these decisions affect the quality and cost of care.

Medicine: The Inexact Science
Unlike exact sciences like physics, medicine is inexact. This is why doctors many times have diverging opinions, sometimes differing dramatically from one another. It is actually not often that doctors agree about the best diagnostic approach and, more importantly, the treatment once a diagnosis is made.

Most decisions made by doctors are not simple; there is usually no clear-cut answer. There are some examples of rare situations in which all doctors agree, such as the case of a patient with a perforated bowel or a patient with bacterial pneumonia. The answer you will get from all doctors in these cases is the same: emergency surgery and appropriate antibiotic, respectively. However, the majority of cases encountered by doctors are not as black and white; they fit in a large and significant area of grey.

Take the example of a 60 year-old patient with chronic lower back pain. Imaging of the patient's lower back (an X-ray and MRI) shows degenerative disc disease of the lumbar spine (essentially, wear and tear of the lower back – a common finding at that age) and a slight degree of pinching of a nerve root. As a doctor, the challenge is to correlate the symptoms, the physical signs upon examination, and the imaging results. It must be determined if the patient's back pain symptoms are caused by the "slight" nerve pinching, the degeneration of the discs itself, the soft tissue inflammation around the degenerated discs, or one of a few other potential issues. Once this is isolated, the best treatment option for the patient is determined, whether that be surgery, physical therapy, medication, or other minimally invasive procedures.

As you can tell, this case, unlike the cases of a perforated bowel and bacterial pneumonia, is very unclear. It, like the majority of cases in medicine, falls into the grey area and is influenced heavily by the "Four Dimensions" of medical decision-making that will be explained later on in this chapter.

The Doctor's Toolbox
Let us start with the basics. Similar to the way we are going about analyzing the U.S. health care system in this book, there are two components of medical management that a medical practitioner must establish: the diagnosis and the treatment.

Of course, the diagnosis is the vital first step because any suggestion of treatment is irrelevant and futile if the first step is faulty. Making a diagnosis involves a three-pronged process:

1. Take the patient's history. This essentially means understanding a patient's symptoms.

2. Examine the patient to elicit physical signs.

The understanding of the patient's symptoms and the elicitation of physical signs by the doctor on examination are together called the "clinical evaluation."

3. Perform diagnostic testing. This testing can include a myriad of tools such as blood testing, imaging, tissue examination, and physiologic testing, among many others.

Except on rare occasions, a doctor cannot make a firm diagnosis by one of the three tools alone. As an example of one of these uncommon situations, a doctor can diagnose some skin diseases by appearance alone, without knowing anything about the symptoms (so only using one prong). The correlation between the three prongs is an important part of arriving at the right diagnosis. They must be taken together to determine if the combination is merely coincidental or actually causative of the patient's symptoms. In an outpatient setting (i.e. a doctor's office), doctors try their best to make a reasonable diagnosis after the clinical evaluation alone, or they do a simple office-based diagnostic test. If this process is not enough to make a reasonably confident diagnosis, testing in a separate facility is needed. In an inpatient setting (i.e. a hospital), all three of the diagnostic tools are necessary and always sought. Even when all three tools are in full effect, in very rare cases, this might not be enough to make a diagnosis, and doctors are left scratching their heads.

I was surprised when I read a few years ago that a radiologist opened a medical center in New York City near Wall Street, hoping to cater to the financial elites and claiming that a "total body scan" can diagnose any hidden diseases. As discussed, a scan is only one of the three tools in the diagnostic process. In the case of this newly opened medical center, there is absolutely no clinical evaluation (the first two diagnostic prongs) to correlate with the scan. You can conclude here that the claim of diagnosing diseases by simply scanning the body is not credible. Even worse, as we will discuss in the next chapter on excessive testing, this may lead to unnecessary, invasive biopsies that can harm a patient or even end a patient's life. These biopsies are all for no good reason! Sound clinical analysis is crucial in ordering tests that are targeted and specific. Otherwise, excessive and unnecessary testing will result, which in itself is costly and may also harm the patient.

The Making and the Making Up of a Doctor's Mind
With this basic understanding, we can now examine what goes into the making of a doctor's mind, which ultimately influences his or her decisions. This can differ from one doctor to another, even as they evaluate the same patient. Our discussion here will shed some light on the subjectivity of the decision-making process and how it influences the economics of health care.

During my time at Ormskirk General Hospital in Lancashire, England, I spent two years in the early 1980s at the post of medical registrar (a hospital-based training job in general medicine, usually attained after at least three years of postgraduate training). In this job, there was a team of four physicians of varying seniority. Every patient admitted to the hospital under general medicine in our department was seen by that team. I was number two in seniority of that four-member team. It was there that I learned the subjectivity of medical decision-making and how medical decisions can vary, sometimes widely. After the four of us would discuss each patient's case and exchange often differing opinions, the root causes of these different opinions took shape. This subjectivity in making medical decisions impacts patients' lives in terms of both quantity and health-related quality. During this period of my training, I conceived the concept of the "Four Dimensions" of the making of a doctor (namely: knowledge, training, experience, and judgment), and it has guided me throughout my professional career. It has helped me to not only strive to give optimal patient service to the best of my abilities, but also to understand and respect my colleagues' views no matter how different they are from my own.

These "Four Dimensions" are the pillars on which a doctor's decision-making process stands. This same concept will be used throughout this book as we reference the inner workings of a doctor, which has relevance to both the outcomes of medical and surgical intervention and the costs to the system.

The First Three Dimensions of the "Making of a Doctor"
To explain the "making of a doctor," one should know that there are three sources of information, or dimensions, a physician considers. Together with a lesser-known "Fourth Dimension" that we will explore later, these sources of information are what determines a physician's decisions.

> *The First Dimension - Knowledge*: The first dimension is the physician's medical schooling. This dimension is shaped by the authors of the textbooks from which aspiring physicians study and the opinions held by their professors.
>
> *The Second Dimension - Training*: The second dimension is the physician's hands-on training through postgraduate residency and fellowship training programs. Besides the training itself, a doctor is growing his or her "knowledge" dimension in this stage also, but with a narrower scope and

more depth than in the first dimension. This phase is crucial because it is the young doctor's first exposure to what the practice of medicine looks like in action. It is in this phase that the young doctor (Resident or Fellow) is trained in evaluating patients and the decision-making process. Young doctors are also trained on how to perform practical actions like surgeries and procedures. Again, and to perhaps a greater degree, the mind of a doctor is shaped by the experience and opinion of his or her teachers and trainers.

The Third Dimension - Experience: The third dimension is the physician's own experience as an independent practitioner. This particular dimension tends to change over one's professional lifetime as a doctor. I have often likened a doctor's professional journey to a color spectrum. On one end of the spectrum, the color red represents the fresh, young doctors who have recently acquired their knowledge during schooling and residency and fellowship training. I refer to this group as "red hot and ready to act." In his or her early years of practice, a young physician often has solutions readily available "within his or her prescription pad," while a young surgeon often has solutions readily available "at the tip of his or her scalpel." Over the years, these doctors acquire wisdom through experience, which is represented by the color blue. Doctors discover that they can actually leave patients worse off with medical and/or surgical intervention than they would have been without it, as we will see in Chapter 13. The optimal doctors are the "purple" doctors – those who have a command of the necessary medical knowledge and training, but have also become wise through experience.

These three sources of information are what make up the mind of a doctor in terms of the knowledge, training, and experience that enters into the decision-making process. It is easy to see how variations in these three dimensions can lead to variations in the decision-making process from doctor to doctor. Differences in schooling, training, and experience create different mindsets.

The Little-Known "Fourth Dimension"
The three factors discussed above that shape the mind of a doctor cause some degree of variation. Now, as the doctor moves into the act of making decisions for his or her patient, there is even more variability and subjectivity. Critically, there is a fourth factor, or dimension, that is far less known. Two doctors could theoretically have the same exact composition of their first three dimensions, yet still come to recommend different treatments for the same patient because of their differing "Fourth Dimension." This dimension shapes the decision-making process, both in terms of deciding on diagnostic tests and, more importantly, in deciding on treatments.

This Fourth Dimension is in some ways analogous to the fourth dimension of space. The three almost universally known dimensions in space are length, width, and depth. The fourth dimension, first introduced by mathematicians in the late 18th and 19th centuries, is time. This fourth dimension is far less understood and talked about than the preceding three, and you almost have to be a mathematician to even know much about it. Similarly, the Fourth Dimension of medical decision-making is scarcely known, and you have to be a doctor to deeply understand it. But I will explain it here as clearly as I can.

> *The Fourth Dimension - Judgment*: The comparable fourth and much lesser-known factor in the realm of medical decision-making – what contributes crucially to the making and the making up of the doctor's mind – is a doctor's personal assessment of risk versus benefit. This is a part of who the doctor is as a person; it is a personality trait that determines a doctor's tendency to take risks or to be cautious. It is a doctor's judgment. This is a dimension that is independent of the other three dimensions, though it is partly influenced by the third dimension over time.

To be sure, the third dimension – a doctor's experience as an independent practitioner – can influence the fourth dimension to a certain extent. Experience tends to temper the tendency to take excessive risk. After discovering over years that certain outcomes by aggressive medical or surgical intervention actually lead to worse results than the initial ailment itself, even the most risk-seeking types will become conservative in their decision-making as they mature as practitioners. As mentioned, physicians or surgeons in their younger years tend to be activists and interventionists. Over years of practice, many of these doctors become less activist in their approach to making medical decisions as they learn that their actions – medical or surgical – may sometimes harm patients more than their inaction. The interventionist approach as a young physician or surgeon is tempered over time. This is simply a trend I have noticed, but it does not hold for all doctors, of course. The old adage attributed to Eleanor Roosevelt rings true here: "Learn from the mistakes of others. You can't live long enough to make them all yourself."

Still, the Fourth Dimension persists beyond the experience factor. Individuals who tend to take excessive risk to start with will continue to do so even if experience partially tempers this instinct. Similarly, but on the opposite end of the spectrum, individuals who are already cautious will continue to be cautious, perhaps even more so, with experience in seeing outcomes of their actions that are more harmful than inaction would have been. This is an overview of how the Fourth Dimension comes into play when doctors make their decisions. Now let us look at some examples.

Real Life Cases Illustrating the "Fourth Dimension" in Action
Here are three real life examples that will help better explain this Fourth Dimension and how it works. I know the first case directly and the other two indirectly, as they were not my patients.

1. *We can start with a female patient - let us call her Alexandra. Alexandra was visiting Jacksonville, and she had a relatively harmless condition called venous insufficiency. It caused swelling of her legs upon*

being upright for a prolonged period of time. So, Alexandra's health care provider prescribed her a powerful diuretic (water pill) called Furosemide (or Lasix). However, normal treatment of these symptoms is not a diuretic (let alone such a powerful one as this, which depletes the body of potassium, a vital element for the body). Rather, if there is no surgically treatable cause for the disorder, regular treatment would simply be frequent elevation of the legs and elastic stockings. Upon taking the pill, Alexandra was found to have very low levels of potassium and consequently had to take additional pills to replenish the potassium in her body that had been lost as a result of the water pill. When I met Alexandra, she was coming to my office with acute abdominal pain, which was found to be due to the perforation of her bowel from the potassium pill that she started taking two days before (a rare occurrence but a known side effect). She had to have emergency surgery to save her life. As you can see, Alexandra was far, far worse off because of the treatment than she would have been without it. And the correct treatment of her illness was actually far simpler – and less expensive – than the one that was given.

2. *The second case is that of a male teenager who saw a doctor with the hope of improving his acne and developing clearer skin. The teenager was given an oral medication called Accutane to treat his acne. After taking the medication for a few weeks, he was found to have committed suicide. Suicidal thoughts are a recognized side effect of Accutane, which was a common treatment for acne until it was discontinued as a regular prescription drug in 2009 (it is still available, but under restricted conditions). Indeed, Accutane was one of the top 10 drugs in the FDA database in terms of the number of reports of depression and suicide attempts among its users.[1] Accutane also has other harmful side effects like pseudotumor cerebri, a condition in which the pressure inside the skull increases and can even blind young patients if left untreated.*

3. *The third case is that of a 41 year-old woman who came to a physician because of a toenail fungal infection. This woman was given an oral antifungal treatment for the infection that is normally taken for several*

months. Later, she tragically died of acute liver failure as a consequence of the oral treatment.

The examples illustrate that even though these treatment modalities for these conditions are common, they are still associated with rare occurrences of serious adverse outcomes. None of the original ailments in these cases (venous insufficiency, acne, and toenail fungal infection) are fatal to patients or even very serious. Treating diseases that never kill patients with a treatment modality that has inherent potential to injure or even kill patients is not sound judgment. This risk-versus-benefit analysis is what the Fourth Dimension is all about. The judgment will never be looked at as unsound if there is no adverse outcome or if there is a mild, reversible adverse outcome of the treatment, which is typically the case. However, it becomes obvious in retrospect if the rare serious or fatal adverse outcome occurs, as in the three aforementioned cases. These are not considered to be malpractice cases because they do not satisfy the legal criteria to make them such, so the onus and responsibility falls on the doctor and his or her judgment. For the doctor, it comes down to essentially weighing a definite zero percent chance of death from the actual diseases in the three examples with a definite greater-than-zero chance of death from the choice of the modalities of treatment. It comes down to the doctor's judgment – his or her Fourth Dimension.

The Four Dimensions, Primary Care, and the Role of "Physician Extenders"
Each of the Four Dimensions is extremely important in medical management, both in making a diagnosis and in suggesting a treatment. Taken together, these four factors are creatures of an inexact science. Operating in the field of primary care, it is easy for me to see how crucial these Four Dimensions are on a regular basis. As the first line of defense in one's medical care, a primary care physician is the gatekeeper for the rest of the health care system. His or her original diagnosis, as well as further diagnostic work or specialist referrals, is critical to the outcome of the patient's care. The primary care physician must have an ideal combination of

knowledge, training, experience, and judgment to be able to make the correct decisions on a daily basis. There is simply too much riding on our decisions to take this lightly.

So, in understanding the mind of a doctor, we can see how this might differ from other health care providers. Nurse practitioners and physician assistants (a group together called "physician extenders"), for example, have been taking more significant roles as of late. The advent of this category of health care providers may seem, on the surface, to be a way to cut costs. Indeed it does in terms of salaries, but these physician extenders can actually contribute a great deal to the total increase in health care costs. Let us consider this category of health care providers in terms of the core three dimensions. In the case of physician extenders, 1) The First Dimension is not uniformly structured and is suboptimal when compared to the education of a physician, 2) The Second Dimension is minimal, and 3) There are generally fewer chances to develop a Third Dimension, as there is limited experience gained through independent decision-making, since physician extenders normally work under the supervision of a licensed doctor.

Now, we can see how the costs can actually be increased when physician extenders are given a lot of the decision-making responsibility that physicians used to hold. Most of the cost of health care in the primary care setting hinges on referrals to specialists, diagnostic testing, and overprescribing. Due to physician extenders' lack of depth of knowledge and training when compared to a physician, there is a higher tendency to both refer patients to specialists and test excessively. So, it is my opinion that physician extenders are best utilized in a specialist setting, where they can be quite valuable, not in a primary care setting.

SECTION II.
THE DIAGNOSIS: PAYING MORE

With this broad-scale understanding of the problems facing our national health care system, as well as a look into the minds of physicians who make the all-important decisions about our health, we can move on to a "diagnosis" of the problem. We have a very clear problem of paying a lot to get a little – there is no argument there. But with such a large problem that so deeply affects hundreds of millions of lives, how do we begin to delve into the components of that problem, analyzing it piece-by-piece to get to solutions?

In this section of the book, we will start by diagnosing the "paying more" portion of the problem. To do this, we will divide up this part of the problem into components: those that are caused primarily by the medical profession (excessive testing, doctors overprescribing, bypassing the primary care physician, physicians not assessing costs to system, and – later on – costs related to iatrogenic diseases) and those that are caused by other factors (waste caused by insurance and billing companies, overpriced pharmaceuticals and medical devices, a fragmented hospital system, ever-increasing administrative costs for medical offices, and direct-to-consumer marketing by pharmaceutical companies).

Throughout this diagnosis, keep in mind that there is an underlying thread of three aspects of the system that continue to plague it: it is expensive, it is fragmented, and it is inefficient.

SECTION II, PART A:
COSTS CAUSED PRIMARILY BY THE MEDICAL PROFESSION

CHAPTER FOUR
EXCESSIVE TESTING

We will begin with excessive testing by doctors. As we will see, excessive testing is costly both in that it is very expensive and – more importantly – in that it can injure or even kill a patient!

Causes of Excessive Testing
There are several different reasons for why excessive testing has become such a mammoth problem in the American health care system. I will outline a few of them here.

1. Faulty Clinical Analysis
The process by which a physician or surgeon analyzes his or her patient clinically (from symptoms and examination only) is crucial in planning a diagnostic work-up that is specific and targeted. If this analysis is done well, there is a higher chance of reaching an accurate diagnosis with minimal testing. However, this clinical analysis, when it is not sound, can lead to excessive and unnecessary testing. In primary care, the diagnostic work-up is far more complex than in a specialist setting. Primary care physicians deal with the whole body, so the diagnostic process is accordingly vast. A specialist, on the other hand, has a narrow field of specialty and thus has limited diagnostic tests to consider. Ensuring a targeted and specific diagnostic work-up requires sound clinical analysis, which is a function of the "Four Dimensions" that make up a doctor. These Four Dimensions, as you recall, are knowledge, training, experience, and judgment.

The less a provider of health care has of these Four Dimensions, the more tests are ordered, and vice versa, especially in the field of primary care. This is so solid of a fact that both the two opposing systems of health care I experienced (the public system in the U.K. and the mostly private system in the U.S.) agree on it. Each system uses different methods to safeguard against the ordering of expensive testing. In the U.S., insurance companies outsource this safeguarding process to the National Imaging Association (NIA). Essentially, a physician – most likely a radiologist – calls the doctor ordering the expensive test (usually an imaging scan) and they confer together. Even though this conferring is useful, it is asymmetrical. The radiologist is trained in radiology and makes opinions as far as the best imaging test available for the suspected diagnosis (and has the often-used authority to deny the test if the treating doctor does not make a strong case), but the treating doctor is a clinician trained in analyzing patients through taking history and making examinations. As you can deduce from this, it is impossible to find a substitute for a good clinician (treating doctor) with a solid Four Dimensions to ensure that expensive tests are justifiably ordered.

2. Fear of Malpractice

There is no doubt that personal injury and medical malpractice lawyers are partly behind excessive testing by doctors. Medical malpractice lawyers cause excessive testing by incentivizing the doctor to over-test a patient so that he or she can be entirely sure that he or she will not be sued. If a potentially serious diagnosis is an extremely remote possibility but ends up being the case, and it could possibly be blamed on a lack of testing, the malpractice attorneys will have a field day. In many ways, these lawyers took the common sense out of the practice of medicine; they cripple a doctor's better judgment. The common sense approach to thinking through possible diagnoses involves considering probabilities and likelihoods in light of the particular clinical presentation.

There is a wise saying in our profession: "common diseases are encountered more often." If a patient presents to a doctor with a headache, the doctor does not test for a brain tumor (except in rare cases when that is indicated from clinical evaluation) because there are far more common causes of headaches. In the eyes of a malpractice lawyer, however, this common sense approach is not valid, and every test for every disease should be done no matter how rare the disease may be!

Measuring just how much of the cost of excessive testing should be blamed on the malpractice law environment is challenging. This is partly because doctors at times rationalize excessive testing for other reasons and merely use the excuse of seeking to avoid malpractice laws. Though it is difficult to quantify, this fear of malpractice plays a significant role for certain. In one study published by the National Institute of Health (NIH), it was found that overall annual medical liability system costs, including defensive medicine, were estimated to be $55.6 billion in 2008, or 2.4 percent of total health care spending at the time.[1]

Additionally, the actual system of hearing malpractice cases creates undue liability for doctors. This is because trial attorneys can and often do take advantage of the complexity of statistics and the lack of knowledge about medicine among the jurors to unfairly sway them to the side of the plaintiff. As a juror, one is likely to have trouble seeing beyond the injured patient testifying before him or her and is unlikely to be able to navigate the complexity of the case. As we will discuss in the "treatment" section, there is certainly a need for reform in this arena.

3. Greed

Yes, greed does exist among doctors, even though it may be rare. Doctors are human beings and members of society just like all other people. They are like any other sect of society; the vast majority are good, but very occasionally there are the evil and self-serving. As an example, fee-for-service (FFS) reimbursement, the most dominant method of physician payment in the United States, can sometimes misincentivize doctors.[2] In FFS, all services provided by a physician are unbundled, and payers reimburse the physician a certain amount for each procedure. This structure can inadvertently put more emphasis on quantity of care rather than quality of care. One of the ironies of how this FFS system works is that the "level of service" rendered when a patient sees a doctor is higher when more tests are ordered, regardless of whether the tests are done in-house or referred to outside facilities. The more tests that are ordered, the higher the payment for that visit.

There have been attempted safeguards against some self-serving practices, such as the Stark Law, which prohibits doctors from referring to imaging facilities or laboratories if the doctor has a financial relationship with that entity. However, it crucially does not safeguard against diagnostic procedures performed by the doctors themselves.

4. Lack of Communication Between Providers: A Fragmented System
A good deal of excessive testing is due to the fragmented nature of health care. Quite often, a physician or hospital will repeat a test that another physician or hospital has already completed without the two providers knowing about one another. Unifying the Electronic Health Record (EHR) platform is a part of the solution here, as we will discuss in the "treatment" section later on. When a patient comes to a primary care physician's office with a prior visit to a hospital or two and one specialist or more, it is currently virtually impossible logistically to track all the information from these providers to view results and avoid duplicate testing. Unfortunately, we in the medical profession do not live in an interconnected world (yet), though patients expect us to. The good news, as we will discuss, is that this problem of "fragmented medicine" is relatively easy to treat.

5. Testing Begets More Testing (and may harm or kill the patient along the way)
In a normal, healthy human being there are sometimes "abnormal" test results, whether it is on a blood test, an imaging report, or a physiologic test. These abnormal results can be benign and occur in perfectly healthy individuals, so they must be carefully considered in light of the other clinical findings and information

about the patient. The presence of these test results will often cause additional tests to be done, whether due to the physician's fear of liability or lack of experience. In other words, testing often begets more testing. At times, adverse health outcomes – sometimes even death – result from the process of conducting these tests, particularly if they are invasive in nature.

Examples of "Testing Begets More Testing"
Let us consider some examples to illustrate that excessive testing causes more excessive testing:

> 1. First, let us consider Irritable Bowel Syndrome (IBS), a motility dysfunction affecting the digestive system and large bowel in particular. It causes abnormal bowel movement, with symptoms ranging from diarrhea to constipation to an alternation of both, among other digestive symptoms. IBS is caused by emotional stress; there is no underlying physical disease. One in ten people globally, mostly women, suffer from IBS.[3] There are even some estimates suggesting that this disorder is more common, affecting as many as one in seven people. There is no test to confirm IBS; it is essentially a presumptive diagnosis. It is important to note that IBS is not necessarily a diagnosis of exclusion (a diagnosis of exclusion is one that can only be made by the process of elimination). This means that it is generally not necessary to conduct several tests in order to make a presumptive diagnosis of IBS. However, many doctors order many tests and make their diagnosis of IBS based on these tests coming back negative. Essentially, the diagnosis is not made based on what is found in these tests but rather what is NOT found!
>
> Quite often, patients leave the gastroenterologist's office with a diagnosis of IBS, but many undergo upper gastrointestinal endoscopies and colonoscopies (procedures to visualize the upper and lower digestive tract) first. Patients may also end up having imaging of the

abdomen done (like a CAT scan or MRI) because of the abdominal pain that is often a symptom of the disorder. These and other extraneous tests are ordered by a doctor in an attempt to avoid overlooking other conditions, but they are often unnecessary. Additionally, there are a host of coincidental abnormalities that occur in perfectly healthy patients within abdominal solid organs like the liver, pancreas, spleen, kidneys, and adrenal gland. So, when these innocuous abnormalities are noticed in the midst of the barrage of tests, the result is the doctor ordering unnecessary, invasive biopsies, which can harm the patient or even end his or her life.

Instead of conducting all of these tests, a prudent primary care physician may find the age of onset of symptoms (typically young), duration of symptom (typically long), and absence of other lab abnormalities (blood tests and stool analysis) to be sufficient to make a reasonable, presumptive diagnosis of IBS, while sparing the patient and the system unnecessary, expensive, and potentially harmful testing.

2. A second example involves the nuclear stress test of the heart, which is used to diagnose coronary artery disease (CAD). CAD is a disease of the arteries that supply the heart muscle with blood, which can lead to a heart attack. At least 20 percent of stress tests with imaging yield either a false positive (meaning the test suggests the presence of a condition that is in fact not present) or a false negative (meaning the test suggests the absence of a condition that is in fact present) for the diagnosis of CAD.[4] Following any positive nuclear stress test, an invasive cardiac catheterization is often performed, which has an inherent risk of death, albeit a small one. Any resulting harm is due to the invasive test (which may be negative) that was done as a result of a possibly false positive yielded by the initial test. The invasive test would not have been performed in

the first place if the nuclear stress test had not been done. This is an unspeakable error and the potential for these mistakes grows exponentially as more testing is undergone.

The cause of anterior chest pain in a patient presenting to a primary care physician in an outpatient setting is far more likely to be a non-cardiac one. There are several other causes of such pain. Consideration of the presence or absence of risk factors for coronary artery disease – in conjunction with sound clinical analysis and careful consideration of some other more common, non-cardiac causes for the chest pain – is the correct way forward; this would steer the doctor away from initiating all of the aforementioned tests.

It takes an experienced physician with a strong set of Four Dimensions to avoid these types of testing pitfalls. As we will discuss in the "treatment" section, it is paramount that primary care physicians are well-trained to avoid initiating these cycles of over-testing.

Real Life Cases of "Testing Begets More Testing"
Now let us consider two more personal examples to illustrate the concept that "testing begets more testing." These two examples were not my patients, but I knew of their situations indirectly.

1. *A healthy woman in her mid-forties had a CAT scan of the abdomen ordered by her doctor to assess her pancreas. The abdominal CAT scan as reported by the radiologist showed a nodule, which was later confirmed to be an adenoma (a harmless, not uncommon finding in a perfectly healthy patient) in the adrenal gland (an endocrine gland located above the kidneys). This finding was coincidental and had nothing to do with the initial reason for ordering the test. Though some adenomas can occasionally be functional (i.e. secrete hormones abnormally), this problem can be detected by blood and/or urine testing. The doctor recommended a biopsy, which sadly involved intra-abdominal bleeding (bleeding inside the abdominal cavity). Ultimately,*

the woman had to have emergency surgery to save her life! Thankfully, she lived through the surgery. In the end, the biopsy showed that the nodule was in fact a non-functioning adenoma, which is a benign condition posing no risk to patients!

2. *A woman in her early fifties who is a non-smoker — let's call her Joanne — saw her primary care provider (a physician extender saw her) with complaints of coughing. She had a chest X-ray which happened to show a very small "spot" (a quite common observation due to various benign findings such as scar tissue, among other things). Her primary care provider continued to check on the spot on her chest X-ray for four years by repeating a CAT scan of her lungs. Most doctors will probably agree that following up on a very small spot on the lung for four years in the case of a patient with no smoking history is excessive and unnecessary. It should have been followed up on only once in a reasonable timespan of three to six months to make sure it was not growing. If a spot like this does not grow in this timespan, it can be presumed to be caused by something benign, like a scar; there is then no need for further follow-up because scars do not become cancerous over time.*

After four years of follow-up imaging, the radiologist thought the spot "may be getting larger" and attempted a percutaneous transpleural lung biopsy (using a wide bore needle through the skin under CAT scan guidance). This failed, so he decided to send Joanne to a pulmonologist (a lung specialist). The pulmonologist tried to get a biopsy through bronchoscopy (visualizing airways) to see if he could reach the spot to be biopsied, but failed.

As a last resort, Joanne was sent to a thoracic surgeon, who did a thoracotomy (incision into the chest through cutting ribs). This is a direct approach to the lung. It also involved difficult manipulation of the lung to reach the spot shown on the chest imaging. Sadly, there was a complication during this procedure. Joanne ended up in an intensive care unit. To add insult to this very avoidable injury, the pathology report eventually showed that the spot, which had not been growing after all, was merely scar tissue.

In an intensive care unit, one is teetering between life and death. Anything can go wrong, and any slight problem can be deadly. Thankfully, Joanne lived on and made it out of the intensive care unit. However, the result was easily hundreds of thousands of dollars of wasted medical expenses and physical as well as emotional scars to match.

The two healthy patients above could have easily died because of the cycle of testing that began with a coincidental abnormality that was eventually deemed innocuous. As we will see, there is an immense economic cost generated when doctors cause greater health problems due to excessive testing as well as unnecessary surgeries and invasive procedures.

Ultimately, the fact that these patients lived does not erase the financial, emotional, and physical turmoil that came from the performance of unnecessary additional testing. Indeed, excessive testing is real and is hurting our citizens and our nation as a whole in all three aspects of health – financial, physical, and emotional.

CHAPTER FIVE
DOCTORS OVERPRESCRIBING

In addition to this problem of doctors over-testing, there is the issue of doctors overprescribing. Medical students study the field of pharmacology (the study of drugs and their actions) in the early stages of their medical schooling. Learning to write prescriptions is easy and is perhaps most symbolic of a core "doctor-like action." While the act of writing prescriptions is one of the first skills studied as a young doctor or physician extender, it takes time in practice to realize that excessive prescribing is not only an unhealthy practice economically, but it also can be a physically harmful or even lethal practice.

A Proliferation of Prescription Drug Use and a Troubling Trend
Prescription drug use in the United States is incredibly common. A 2014 IMS Institute analysis found that on average, Americans – including those who are healthy and untreated – use 12.2 prescriptions per year.[1] According to a CDC report, from 2007 to 2010 almost one-half of all Americans reported taking one or more prescription drugs in the past 30 days. The rate of usage increased with age, going from one in four children to 9 in 10 persons aged 65 and over.[2]

The recent trends are particularly stunning and a bit frightening. Prescription drug use in the U.S. has been on a dramatic rise in recent decades, particularly the last 20 years. According to a 2010 Kaiser Foundation report, the number of prescriptions in the U.S. increased 39 percent (from 2.8 billion to 3.9 billion) from 1999 to 2009, compared to U.S. population growth of nine percent. The same study found that the average number of retail prescriptions per person was 12.6 in 2009 (a similar conclusion to the aforementioned IMS analysis), which is a significant increase from the 10.1 prescriptions per person just a decade earlier.[3] The CDC National Center for Health Statistics (NCHS) Data Brief published in 2010 found that between 1999 and 2008, the percentage of Americans who took at least one prescription drug in the past month increased from 44 percent to 48 percent.[4] Interestingly, many drugs that used to require a prescription are now available over-the-counter, such as treatments for allergies, acid-reflux, and other conditions. One would think that the effectiveness of these medications and the commonality of the conditions they treat would actually be factors that *reduce* the number of prescription drugs significantly, but that is clearly not the overall trend we are seeing here.

It is also worth mentioning that if a new drug or class of drugs enters the market, it essentially replaces the older drugs that used to be prescribed for that same disease. So, this should not be a factor in the recent increase in prescriptions per person.

Increase in Prescription Narcotic Use
Recent decades have also seen a dramatic increase in the number of prescriptions for narcotics (opium derivatives). According to the CDC, health care providers wrote 259 million prescriptions for painkillers in 2012, which is shockingly enough for every American adult to have a bottle of pills.[5]

Making comparisons internationally is even more striking. The U.S. has twice as many painkiller prescriptions per person as Canada.[6] Though only 4.6 percent of the world's population, Americans have been consuming 80 percent of the global opioid (a semi-synthetic opium derivative) supply.[7] Prescriptions for opiates (opium derivatives) have escalated from around 40 million in 1991 to nearly 180 million in 2007, with the U.S. as the biggest consumer.[8] According to the CDC, the consumption of opioid analgesics pain relievers increased 300 percent between 1999 and 2010, and death rates for associated poisoning more than tripled between 2000 and 2010.[9]

This increase in the availability of these prescription painkillers has also led to an increase in abuse and overdose. We in the state of Florida have a huge epidemic of this, even though the problem has improved after legislation implemented in 2010 and 2011. Patients used to come from many other faraway states to get narcotic prescriptions from Florida, a practice coined as "narco-tourism" by journalists. The effects are tragic; in 2009, the CDC found that approximately eight deaths due to drug overdose occurred each day in the state of Florida alone, and 76 percent of all drug overdose deaths were related to prescription medications.[10] And this amount of Florida deaths due to narcotics does not include deaths of users who obtained narcotics from Florida and then died after returning to their home states.

Using Multiple Drugs Simultaneously (Polypharmacy)
Not only are more people taking drugs, more people are taking *multiple* drugs at the same time (a practice called polypharmacy). From 2007 to 2010, the CDC found that 13.9 percent of American adults aged 18 and over reported taking five or more drugs in the past 30 days.[11] Other estimates suggest that one-quarter to one-half of U.S. adults aged 65 and older take five or more medications concurrently.[12] The trend over time, as you would expect, is a steep increase; the CDC found that the use of two or more drugs increased from 25 percent to 31 percent from 1999 to 2008.[13] And it is not rare to find that some of these people are taking multiple drugs within the same family of pharmaceuticals.

Polypharmacy exponentially increases the chances of having an adverse reaction and problematic drug interactions, as well as dosing and compliance issues. This is especially true in older populations. In the United States, it is estimated that annually from 2007 to 2009 there were nearly 100,000 emergency hospitalizations for adverse drug events in individuals 65 years and older, with nearly two-thirds due to unintentional overdoses.[14]

The Harm and the Cost

Medicines are mostly foreign chemicals to the human body. Just as a foreign chemical is potentially poisonous to humans, so is medicine. You do not have to be a student of chemistry to know that there are multitudes of toxicities in each drug. As we know, medications often have pernicious side effects. The interactions of multiple medications can be particularly harmful. As mentioned previously, every medication added to the mix not only increases potential side effects and toxicities, but also exponentially increases the likelihood that an interaction between two or more of the drugs being taken will be harmful.

To attempt to further quantify the harm, if it were classified as a disease, adverse drug reactions would by some estimates be between the fourth and sixth leading cause of death in the U.S.[15] Once again, we have an example here in which patients are consuming more health resources and thus increasing costs only to ultimately cause a greater likelihood of harm to themselves. Put simply, we have another example of how we as Americans are paying more to get less.

Seconds to Prescribe, Irreversible Mistakes

Polypharmacy is perhaps the best example of a doctor's poor Fourth Dimension. A doctor with a poor sense of judgment will overprescribe drugs without carefully considering the potential side effects and interactions. It takes seconds to write a new prescription, but it is quite the undertaking to wean patients off of drugs they have been accustomed to taking. Some patients develop physical dependencies, as with narcotics and other non-narcotic addictive drugs, and it is hard to stop these dependencies. Even if a patient is taking a medication that does not cause physical dependency, he or she may develop a psychological dependency to the drug. Ultimately, then, stopping a patient's use of drugs that can be harmful to them alone or in concert with other drugs is incredibly difficult and sometimes impossible. This is indeed one of the most troublesome challenges in American health care today.

While many drugs have changed health care for the better,

more medication is not necessarily best. It is a very important role for a physician to educate patients and steer them away from the false belief that one can "gobble up medicines on the way to living eternally." In reality, polypharmacy is too frequently the shortest way to the grave, or at least to a significant loss of well-being.

CHAPTER SIX
BYPASSING THE PRIMARY CARE PHYSICIAN: DIRECT-TO-SPECIALIST REFERRALS AND CONSULTATIONS

This is one of the stealthiest causes of health care cost increases, but it is a very important one. Increasing reliance on specialists without the patient being evaluated first by a primary care physician (PCP) is a huge and very consequential practice in terms of health care costs. Whether it is because of direct specialist-to-specialist referrals or direct patient-to-specialist consultations, this practice is not just expensive, but it can also be detrimental to patients. It has the potential of starting the cycle of expensive and potentially harmful (or even lethal) processes described in Chapter 4 as "testing begets more testing."

We should take a moment here and note that the issue of direct patient-to-specialist consultations is not caused by the medical profession; it is rather an issue of patients' choices and insurances allowing patients to consult specialists directly. We only discuss it in this section for convenience as we explore all harmful effects that come from consultations to specialists not initiated by a PCP.

The Role of a Primary Care Physician
To understand the problem with specialist-to-specialist referrals and direct patient-to-specialist consultations, one must first grasp the role of the primary care physician. The PCP is truly at the center of everything in health care.

The primary care physician is the entity in the medical

profession that focuses on the entire body, without specializing in one particular area. Because of this, the PCP is able to see the patient holistically, without having a bias towards a particular region of the body. Conversely, specialists see the patient through the system in which they are trained and experienced. Often, patients will present symptoms – for example, "leg pain" or "chest pain"– that can be caused by a variety of diseases across medical and surgical specialties. Thus, the only entity equipped to make at least a provisional diagnosis is the PCP. The primary care physician makes the original diagnosis and then makes the referral, if necessary, to the appropriate specialist. A specialist can then define and further refine the diagnosis, but this is only after the original diagnosis is made.

The analogy I use to relay this difference is as follows: if a patient is like a tree in a forest, the primary care physician does not see enough detail to see the leaves on the tree, and he or she can make out the branches only hazily. But he or she sees the tree and the overall forest itself very well. The specialist, however, has the opposite perspective. He or she sees the details of the leaves and the branches very well, but only sees the tree hazily and does not see the forest at all. To move even further with the analogy, if there is an environmental problem nearby in the soil next to the tree that will kill it in short order, the specialist will not see that because he or she has such a focused view. The specialist will then assume all is well in the tree (which cannot be fully seen) and will give a clean bill of health to the patient, even though there is real danger lurking nearby.

Put through the lens of another analogy, a specialist looks at the picture of the body through a microscope. He or she analyzes and knows everything about the particular, zoomed-in area at which he or she is looking. The specialist can know the minutest details of that area, but he or she will not see outside the boundaries. In contrast, the PCP looks at a full-body, panoramic picture; he or she can connect and relay one body system to another. While the PCP cannot see the specific details of a particular area, he or she can see how everything connects to each other and how all the systems of the body work together within the patient, who is – after all – a person with a unique physical, emotional, and psychological make-up. The PCP thus has the luxury of a full view.

With this more complete view of the patient, the PCP is relied on to make connections between different problems going on with the patient, address the problems that can be addressed without referring to a specialist, and then refer to the appropriate specialty if and when needed. As the "home base" doctor, the primary care physician is then the one who generally follows up and continues to see the patient in the future. Indeed, the diagnosis and treatment process starts and ends with the primary care doctor.

The PCP's role in health care should never be underestimated.

The Value of a Primary Care Physician

A commentary by Dr. Barbara Starfield of Johns Hopkins University uses a great deal of evidence to show the benefits of strong primary care performance on a country's health system. Dr. Starfield's comparison of 13 countries' health systems across 16 available health indicators showed the United States coming in at an average of 12th place (add this to the running list of studies that put the U.S. far down the list of health care systems in the world). While the reason for this underperformance is multifactorial, it is theorized in Dr. Starfield's article that the lack of a strong primary care infrastructure in our health care system could play a significant role. For example, of the seven countries in the top of the average health rankings, five were considered to have "strong primary care infrastructures."[1] Though better access to care has always been a popular topic of conversation, Dr. Starfield points out that there is evidence showing that "the major benefit of access accrues only when it facilitates the receipt of primary care."[2]

An evidence review by the American College of Physicians (ACP) in 2008 compiled data from 100 medical and scientific documents spanning 20 years of research and concluded that PCPs: reduce mortality rates, reduce unnecessary hospitalizations and emergency room admissions, improve quality and outcomes, provide continuity in health care, reduce overall health care costs and utilization, and are essential to optimal preventive care.[3] Another study led by Dr. Starfield, Dr. Leiyu Shi, and Dr. James Macinko of the Johns Hopkins University Bloomberg School of Public Health cited several possible explanations for why such benefits arise from primary care; they found that effective PCPs provide greater access to needed services, higher quality of care, a greater focus on prevention, early management of health problems, and reduction in unnecessary and potentially harmful specialist care.[4]

Thus, there is substantial and plentiful evidence to support the positive impact of primary care on a health care system. Even within the U.S., states that have higher ratios of primary care physicians to population have better health outcomes, including decreased mortality from cancer, heart disease, or stroke.[5] Yet the U.S. primary care system as a whole ranks very low in comparison to other industrialized countries. And experts project that the U.S. will soon experience a shortage of PCPs, as we will discuss later on.

Direct Specialist-to-Specialist Referrals
Direct referral from a specialist to another specialist is problematic, and direct patient-to-specialist consultation is even worse, both medically and economically. In each case, the PCP is not looped into the consultation, and the situation may not end well. A well-trained PCP is vital in this sense, and we will make sure to discuss the need for improved training of PCPs in a dedicated chapter within the "treatment" section of this book.

Upon hearing this warning about specialist-to-specialist referrals, one may push back. One may think that there is nothing wrong with one specialist referring to another because, after all, specialists are doctors too! They have undergone complete medical training and know about the entire body. While this is correct, the reality is that after 10 to 15 years of practicing in a particular specialty, the doctor will not be too familiar with the rest of the body. As with most things, you lose what you do not use. Indeed, a specialist who has focused on one area for years upon years will likely have far less general medical knowledge than would a final year medical student!

If you do not believe me, quiz your specialist on an area outside of his or her specialty the next time you visit, especially if he or she has been practicing for more than 10 years in that specialty. Ask your urologist if he or she knows that there are 10 layers in the retina of the eye and if he or she can name them. Ask your dermatologist how to treat poorly controlled diabetes. Ask your orthopedic surgeon if he or she knows what diseases affect the adrenal gland. I hope that you see my point. There is no entity better equipped to make an "original diagnosis" like a well-trained PCP. The role of specialists is in defining the diagnosis or refining it further, as well as in treating when deemed appropriate.

Direct Patient-to-Specialist Consultations

As mentioned, direct patient-to-specialist consultation – when a patient goes directly to a specialist and bypasses the primary care physician altogether – has similar and sometimes deeper pitfalls when compared to direct specialist-to-specialist referrals. In either case, the PCP is not looped into the consultation and unnecessary consultations may be made. Though this is not directly caused by doctors, it is a hindrance in ensuring that the primary care physician acts as the "gatekeeper" to the complicated world of health care.

CHAPTER SEVEN
DOCTORS NOT ASSESSING THE COSTS TO THE SYSTEM

This will be the final chapter focusing on the medical profession's role in the "paying more" problem of our health care system. We will be focusing on the issue of the physician's mentality and incentives. It is also a commentary on the societal and medical culture in the United States.

Tendency to Choose Expensive Procedures
Physicians and surgeons often make decisions without regard to evidence-based medicine in light of the magnitude of costs. Because of this, the tendency is to choose more expensive procedures that have less solid evidence of past success.

For example, open-heart surgery is executed far more frequently in the United States than in Canada. A population-based study compared the treatment received by elderly patients who had an acute myocardial infarction (heart attack) in the U.S. versus in Canada. The study found that the U.S. patients are five times more likely to undergo coronary angiography (an invasive procedure to examine the heart blood vessels), almost eight times more likely to undergo percutaneous transluminal coronary angioplasty (a procedure to widen narrowed arteries), and more than seven times more likely to undergo coronary-artery bypass surgery (surgery in which a portion of a healthy vessel is used to create a bypass around the narrowed/ blocked vessel supplying the heart) during the first 30 days after the heart attack. While the study showed that the 30-day mortality rate was slightly lower for the U.S. patients, the one-year mortality rates for the American and Canadian patients were essentially identical – 34.3 percent in the U.S. and 34.4 percent in Ontario.[1] Needless to say, open-heart surgery is extremely expensive and also adds the risk inherent in surgery and anesthesia. An evidence-based cost-benefit analysis must be performed before these invasive procedures are recommended. It seems that this is a cultural issue in the practice of medicine in the U.S.: doctors are not encouraged to weigh the costs and risks of procedures at the level they should. The fee-for-service model used in much of our health care system likely played a role in why the U.S. doctors performed more of these operations than their Canadian counterparts.

Doctors Not Considering the Patient as a "Consumer"
The essence of the issue here is that because doctors do not internalize the costs of these procedures, they are not making decisions that are economically sound. Consider hypothetically if the costs of procedures fell directly to the doctors or the patients. In the case of the previous example of open-heart surgery, the doctor and patient would surely choose not to have the surgery after analyzing the evidence and realizing that the results of the surgery are about the same as the results of the more conservative, cheaper treatment. So, greater consideration of evidence-based information will often decrease costs associated with risky, invasive procedures.

The Problem of Over-Insurance
The problem of expensive, risky procedures is worse when patients are "over-insured," in which case they tend to ask for more, whether necessary or unnecessary. I have had my own experiences with some patients in the past who had more than one insurance plan, so they had no out-of-pocket expenses. For this reason, they wanted excessive testing done. I have had to spend time dissuading them and educating them that they did not need the tests. Because they do not have to pay directly, the "over-insured" may "want it all," and it is a difficult task to inform them that these tests can lead

to added unnecessary tests and can even harm them.

More Expensive Medication Does Not Mean More Effective Treatment
The problem of doctors not considering the cost to the system or to the patient does not stop at surgery and procedures; it also includes the choice of pharmaceuticals. Quite often, there is a drug that is equally as effective, or even more effective, than a newer, better-promoted drug that comes with a much higher ticket price. I have even seen a few examples of medicines that cost tens of times more than equally-effective medicines. Yet these pricier drugs are still prescribed. It should be a training requirement for doctors to spend time learning "health care economics" and how their decisions may be contributing to our system's problems.

SECTION II, PART B:
COSTS CAUSED BY OTHER FACTORS

For the rest of this section (the next five chapters), we will consider cost-raising problems in the health care system that are not caused by the medical profession. In fact, these factors make both patients and doctors alike victims of the other players in the system.

CHAPTER EIGHT
THE HEALTH INSURANCE AND MEDICAL BILLING INDUSTRIES: THE TWO MIDDLEMEN

Accordingly, we can move on from the relatively little-blamed group – physicians – to the group that is probably the most-blamed in every discussion about the problems of American health care, particularly the cost of it: the insurance industry. This industry adds a layer of cost to the system. In my opinion, the inordinate costs involved with the insurance industry are the most glaring area of waste in the system. Out of the difficulty experienced by providers in getting paid by these insurance companies came the need for the medical billing industry, which is yet another unnecessary layer of cost. Thankfully, these two "middlemen" correspond to the easiest of the remedies to present, as we will see in the "treatment" section later on.

Indeed, the costs incurred by the health insurance industry and the medical billing industry are incredibly high, and these costs do not have anything to do with helping to care for patients directly. Let us explore what is going on a bit more closely.

Health Insurance: Profit is the Aim
It will not come as a surprise to anyone that most health insurers are for-profit, publicly-owned entities. Their goal is profit by any means so that they can enrich stockholders. This means profit is often behind their decisions, such as increasing premiums, increasing the out-of-pocket costs that insured patients must pay every time they receive a service, and determining what is allowed or not allowed under the insurance plans.

The Administrative Costs of Health Insurers
Health insurance companies are like a middleman between providers and patients, so their costs should be kept as low as possible as the money is not being used to care for patients directly. Unfortunately, the costs are astronomical. It is estimated that about one quarter of all health care costs in the United States is associated with administration, which is far greater than in other nations.[1] A study conducted decades ago (in 1987) found that between 19.3 percent and 24.1 percent of total spending on health care went to health care administration costs, which came to $400 to $497 per person. Meanwhile, Canadians saw between 8.4 percent and 11.1 percent of health care spending go towards administration. The study found that the U.S. proportion of health care spending consumed by administration alone was at least 117 percent higher in the U.S. than in Canada at the time.[2] More than a decade later, the numbers showed that the size of administrative costs had been growing. In 1999, 31 percent of health care expenditure went towards administration, as compared to 16.7 percent in Canada.[3] A more recent study published in 2010 found that administrative costs accounted for the greatest proportion (39 percent) of health care spending differences between the U.S. and Canada.[4]

In 2006, the McKinsey Global Institute (MGI) found that the U.S. spent almost $650 billion above expected on health care when compared to its peer countries in the OECD, even when adjusting for wealth. MGI found that health care administration costs accounted for $91 billion, or 14 percent, of spending above expected. While part of this spending was found to be due to system structure, redundancies and inefficiencies in the system were also to blame.[5]

Big Banks and Big Health Insurers – More in Common Than Meets the Eye
One simple exercise will help you imagine just how much money goes into the administration of health insurance companies: simply look at the tallest skyscrapers and the biggest buildings across the skylines of any American city, and you will undoubtedly find big banks and – you guessed it – big health care insurance companies.

The quest to enrich health insurance executives and their shareholders is literally impossible not to see.

The similarity does not stop there. Big banks with global operations (so-called "money center banks") and big health insurance companies have massive influence on the government as well. As we know, big banks almost brought the world economy to its knees in 2008 by gambling with savers' money. Taxpayers bailed them out because the banks were deemed "too big to fail." These banks were and are considered "too big to prosecute." Former Attorney General Eric Holder, when asked why he did not prosecute the big banks, admitted in a testimony to a Senate Judiciary Committee in 2013 that indeed they are too big to prosecute, stating that prosecuting these big banks would have "a negative impact on the national economy, perhaps even the world economy." Money center banks like JP Morgan have gotten much larger since 2008, which is why Senator Elizabeth Warren from Massachusetts and many other leaders and common Americans alike can be found ringing the alarm bells, though perhaps to no avail.

The sway that these banks have in influencing the government is certainly a concern, and I think we should also be concerned about the sway that health insurance companies have in Washington. Perhaps this will convince you of the need for alarm: the National Journal's Influence Alley found in 2012 that the major health care lobbying group – America's Health Insurance Plans (AHIP) – was secretly funneling a large amount of money to the U.S. Chamber of Commerce for advertising designed to convince Americans that the Affordable Care Act should be defeated. The amount of money was reported to be a shocking $102.4 million over the span of just 15 months. This was all while negotiating with the White House before publically supporting the bill-now-turned-law.[6]

The influence of big health care insurers and big banks in controlling the government is reminiscent of President Dwight Eisenhower's remarks warning the nation of the influence of the "military-industrial complex." We now have a modern day version of the "military-industrial complex" with perhaps a less clever name: the "big bank-health insurer complex."

The Arcane World of Medical Billing Codes and the Genesis of an Industry
Fifteen years ago, I had never heard of the medical billing business. Today, it is one of the most thriving businesses in the health care industry. Because of how difficult insurance companies have made it for providers to get paid for their services, it has in effect created its own menace: the medical billing companies. If insurance companies are like the middleman in the health care process, medical billing companies are like the "middleman to the middleman" between providers and patients. Medical practice groups and even hospitals can be charged roughly between 6 and 12 percent of net collections for outsourcing a medical billing company to bill health insurance and collect payment for services rendered. Instead of having health insurers as the middleman between payers and providers of services, we now have another middleman in between. As a reader, you may logically say that this cannot be true, but it is. Just imagine how much of your health care dollars are not even spent on your actual health care!

Long gone are the days when medical office staff could handle the billing and collection; the system of insurance has simply become too complex and convoluted. Insurance companies have made it difficult to handle paying claims to the providers on behalf of the insured. In fact, this, along with other huge administrative costs for physicians, is one of the reasons that solo medical practices are becoming a thing of the past. Even big hospital systems now outsource to medical billing companies, as they cannot handle the complexity of medical billing. As a poignant example of the magnitude of this new industry, Duke University Hospital has 900 beds for patients. Now compare this to its *1,300 billing clerks!* Canadian hospitals, for a comparison, do not have nearly the same disproportion.[7] As the complexity of billing and coding increases, the administrative burden for those who provide medical services likewise increases. More personnel are needed to accomplish the same tasks. This administrative component is most certainly a factor in America's exorbitant health care costs.

Not only is the world of medical billing and coding intricate and exceedingly difficult to master, it is also a source of inefficiency. In 2011, the American Medical Association (AMA) found that commercial health insurers had a 19.3 percent claims-processing error rate on average, which the AMA estimates to cost $17 billion annually.[8]

So, another layer of health care expenditure and inefficiency has been created, and none of it has to do with your actual health care.

Taking Care of Patients or "Taking Care of Business"?
My office is a solo practice in Jacksonville, Florida that I have run for the past 27 years. I have always staffed my office with medical assistants (who are trained in patient care) and not medical billing coders (who function as billers). However, because of the factors we have discussed, the percentage of medical billing coders in medical office staffing is becoming higher and higher in offices of all sizes. In late 2011, I joined a primary care physician group affiliated with a large hospital system in the area to utilize its resources for billing and dealing with insurance companies. Most other primary care doctors in the area did the same and joined larger groups, whether hospital-affiliated or independent, for the same reason.

Joining the group meant losing almost all of my independence (which is a privilege I held dearly and one my patients appreciated over my many years of practice). Ironically, even this hospital system eventually resorted to outsourcing its billing after I left it in late 2014 to join a large independent physician group.

Delivering great patient care and running a successful business are certainly not mutually exclusive, but it is indeed a costly challenge to find doctors and staff who excel in both areas. And insurance billing is becoming a bigger and bigger problem by the day, even for large hospital systems. Medical office staffing has now become a balancing act of taking care of patients through medical assistants versus "taking care of business" by hiring medical billing coders. As for myself and all fellow practitioners, we must continue to choose taking care of patients first and foremost. Let the system help us do what we do best as medical professionals: take care of patients.

CHAPTER NINE
OVERLY PRICED PHARMACEUTICALS AND MEDICAL DEVICES: MANUFACTURER PRICE GOUGING AND DECEPTIVE PRACTICES

Price Gouging

Pharmaceuticals and medical devices are sold in the U.S. at far higher prices than abroad. In the health statistics reported by the OECD in 2013, the United States was found to have spent far more on pharmaceuticals per person than any other OECD country – nearly $1,000 per person in 2011.[1] In the U.S., drugs account for 12 percent of overall health care costs and 15 percent of total spending above expected (estimated at $98 billion). The McKinsey Global Institute found that drugs in the U.S. are priced 50 percent higher than those in other countries for equivalent molecules, and branded drugs were found to be 77 percent more expensive on a same-drug basis. When MGI included the impact of the drug mix used in the U.S., it concluded that the U.S. spends over 118 percent more for an average pill than peer OECD countries despite the country's use of more generics (see Figure 9.1 on the following page).[2]

These statistics beg the question: why are drugs so much more expensive in the U.S.? While the answer is not black and white, we will attempt to shed some light on the issue. MGI attributes high U.S. drug spending partly to higher prices and a more expensive drug mix. This more expensive drug mix is partly due to the fact that the U.S. tends to adopt newer drugs one to two years before other countries, and newer drugs command higher prices. Another potential explanation is that because the U.S. is a wealthy nation, the U.S. prices must be higher to subsidize research and development (R&D) for the rest of the world. U.S. spending on marketing and sales also drives up costs. But none of these drivers seem to fully account for the huge gap between pharmaceutical prices in the U.S. versus other comparable countries.[3]

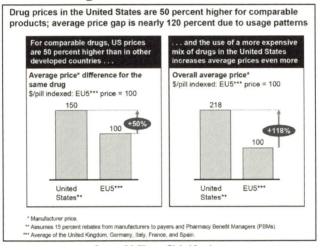

**Figure 9.1
Drug Prices in the United States**

Source: McKinsey Global Institute

How can one explain that the same exact drugs manufactured by the same exact company is sold in Canada (as an example) for far below the prices for which it is sold in the United States? Part of the explanation lies in the U.S.'s lack of negotiating power with drug companies and device manufacturers. No one entity in the U.S. has the power to negotiate prices, whereas Canada does have one such entity (its government). And these companies cannot claim that they are simply "philanthropists" that hope to provide medicine at a lower cost to sub-Saharan African nations and other developing countries. This is clearly false because these companies also sell the medicines at cheaper prices to other Western industrial nations.

Beyond pharmaceuticals, medical devices are also a major source of the expenses of our health care system. There is no doubt that some of these devices improve the quantity and quality of our lives. However, they also may cause serious complications. We as physicians and surgeons should be more proactive in carefully evaluating the pros and cons of any new device, rather than jumping on the bandwagon immediately out of excitement about the novelty and potential of a device. As mentioned before, the fact that the U.S. is an early adopter of almost all forms of new technology is contributing to higher costs.

Certainly, the U.S. should strive to maintain its position as a technological innovator and trailblazer, but perhaps more cost-benefit analyses need to be performed to determine if the increase in costs is worth the added benefit a new drug or device will provide. All that glitters is not gold, and all that is new is not necessarily beneficial. New technologies do not always mean better outcomes. In the worst case scenario, new drugs and devices are sometimes rushed to the market, proven to be harmful, and withdrawn.[4] But this is not without enormous costs shouldered by the system and patients alike. In the case of patients, they would have paid twice: financially through gouged prices and – more significantly – possibly by their own life.

Deceptive Practices
Not only do drug and medical device companies gouge patients in pricing, but they also use deceptive practices at all stages of bringing a drug or device to market. They use clinical trials largely funded by themselves to present to the Food and Drug Administration (FDA) for approval. When a company creating a drug or device sponsors a study to help determine whether or not it will be permitted to go to market, one can reasonably suspect that the results may be compromised. The drug or device may eventually be proven ineffective or harmful and pulled from the market, but – again – only after potentially inflicting harm or death to patients.

Elaborating on the faulty nature of a good deal of clinical research today, Dr. Marcia Angell, former chief editor of *The New England Journal of Medicine* – one of the most renowned medical journals in the world – and current senior lecturer at Harvard Medical School, wrote in 2009, "It is simply no longer possible to believe much of the clinical research that is published."[5] Dr. Richard Horton, the current editor-in-chief of *The Lancet*, another one of the world's most respected medical journals, echoed these statements in an editorial published in *The Lancet* in April 2015 with the title "Offline: What is Medicine's 5 Sigma?" In this article, Dr. Horton states,

> "The case against science is straightforward: much of the scientific literature, perhaps half, may simply be untrue. Afflicted by studies with small sample sizes, tiny effects, invalid exploratory analyses, and flagrant conflicts of interest, together with an obsession for pursuing fashionable trends of dubious importance, science has taken a turn towards darkness."[6]

This is troubling because of the fact that so many medical studies are industry-sponsored, funded from the same accounts that are used to develop drugs, vaccines, and medical devices supposedly to help patients. If the chief editors of arguably the two most prestigious medical publications in the world doubt the accuracy of much of the clinical research out there, there will be no other source to be believed! Money from drug and medical device manufacturers plays a partial but definite role in affecting clinical research outcomes and we all, not just those of us in the medical community, should be extremely concerned.

Digging further into the deceptive practices of drug companies, Dr. Angell authored a 2004 book titled *The Truth About the Drug Companies: How They Deceive Us and What to Do About It*. In this book, Dr, Angell refutes the argument that high drug prices are needed for funding research and discusses how drug companies spend enormous amounts of their money instead in marketing their products, which often do not provide much benefit. Dr. Angell also decries the influence of these companies on the government and, again, on academia.

As pointed out by Dr. Angell, some drug and device companies also uses deceptive methods of advertising their products to patients and doctors alike. To build on this point, Dr. John Abramson, a lecturer at Harvard Medical School, authored a book in 2004 with the title *Overdosed America: The Broken Promise of American Medicine*. This book is an indictment of these companies and their corrupt practices contributing to the commercialization of health care. We will further explore the concept of direct-to-consumer pharmaceutical advertising in Chapter 12.

Between the high prices charged by drug and device companies and the unhealthy influence of these companies on clinical research and government, there is a great deal that needs to be fixed in this area of health care. And many experts agree on this.

CHAPTER TEN
A FRAGMENTED HOSPITAL SYSTEM WITH HIGH OVERHEAD COSTS

Hospitals share less of the blame related to high health care costs even though they are responsible for a significant portion of health care bills. Hospitals are victims of the very high cost of medical technology they must adopt. Expensive diagnostic equipment, especially imaging equipment and advanced technology tools like robotic surgery, is behind these high costs. Even though these very high overhead expenses are passed on to patients and their insurances, these hospitals sometimes do not survive financially. In the last 20 years, I have seen four hospitals in my area of Northeast Florida close their doors as fully-functioning facilities shortly after being acquired by another hospital.

    The following discussion is not about the factors that cause hospitals to have high overhead expenses or how they can cut costs; that is beyond the scope of this book. Rather, it is a discussion of the fragmented hospital system as a part of the overall increase in health care costs, including excessive testing and very high expenses associated with adopting technology. This in turn increases the costs of hospitalization, and these massive costs trickle down to insurance companies and indirectly to the insured through high premiums and co-insurance. Of course, it only takes one hospitalization for an uninsured or underinsured patient to have to spend a lifetime paying the bill, if at all possible, or end up in bankruptcy.

A Fragmented System with Poor Communication
Quite often, patients receive treatment by different providers, either in outpatient or inpatient facilities. The care received by each provider is often not integrated or coordinated; it is fragmented. As we have discussed, this tends to cause redundant testing because the results of a test done in one facility by one physician is not readily available for another physician at another location. This also leads to incomplete and incomprehensive patient health information, which could have serious consequences for the patient if critical pieces of information are not communicated to all providers. Fragmentation leads to inefficient use of resources, higher costs, and at times worse outcomes.

I once saw a patient who had abdominal pain and visited the ER of three different hospitals (each belonging to a different hospital system) within an eight mile radius of my office with the same complaint over the course of four weeks. Each hospital had no way of knowing about the visits to the other hospitals. For whatever reason, the patient did not reveal the other hospital visits to any of the hospital ERs, so each hospital proceeded with needless, repetitive, expensive testing. A large battery of tests, as you may expect, were done on this particular patient at each hospital, and there was considerable overlap in the testing. As it turns out, the patient was insured by Medicaid with no out-of-pocket expenses, but the expenses were still incurred by the system.

Electronic Health Records: A Solution?
In an attempt to help fix these communication issues, the Affordable Care Act mandated Electronic Health Records in place of all paper records. This was meant to help fix the problem of duplicate services in health care.

In theory, adopting EHR technology has enormous potential to increase efficiency, safety, and overall quality of care. However, in practice, EHR is not yet the uniform, integrated, universal database that would generate such gains. The platform of EHR differs from one hospital to another. Putting health records in an electronic format is important, notwithstanding the decrease in physician productivity, but we will have to have a unified platform to reap the full benefits of going electronic. Currently, it is impossible for a physician or a hospital to transfer health records to another physician or hospital with a different software program for EHR. Numerous incompatible platforms of electronic medical records make it difficult and extremely time-consuming to reconcile records. This lack of unification will be discussed further in the latter half of the book, within the "treatment" section.

An example of a successfully integrated EHR system is found within the Veterans Health Administration (VHA). The VHA hospitals and clinics all use a computerized patient record system (CPRS). Initiated in 1994 and implemented nationally in 1999, CPRS allows any provider to access records, tests, labs, and more from any other department or provider within the VHA system, because it is all entered into the patient's health record. When a provider puts in an order for a drug, CPRS has a feature that alerts doctors to any applicable drug contraindications (cases in which a drug should not be used because it may be harmful to the patient) or any potential interactions that may occur with a drug that the patient is already taking. In addition, it alerts the doctor if the patient has an allergy to the drug or if this drug is already being taken by the patient, and so forth. The system also has a component that puts reminders in the patient's record, alerting providers when the patient is due for a flu shot, diabetic eye exam, and so on.[1] Not only does this decrease human error and improve quality of care, but it also reduces waste. One study found that since its full nation-wide implementation in 1999, the CPRS system helped increase the VHA health care system's productivity by almost 6 percent each year.[2] When compared with the Medicare fee-for-service program, the VHA performed significantly better on all 11 overlapping quality indicators for the period from 1997 through 1999, and in 2000 the VHA outperformed Medicare on 12 of 13 overlapping indicators.[3]

EHR has the potential to dramatically change our health care system for the better, but only when it is uniform, integrated, and comprehensive will the maximum benefits be realized.

CHAPTER ELEVEN
EVER-INCREASING ADMINISTRATIVE COSTS FOR MEDICAL PRACTICES

While hospitals may have the resources to survive with the new EHR requirements (though the costs do significantly affect them), medical offices are not in such a position. Between EHR and complex changes to the diagnosis classification system, medical practices are finding it extremely difficult to cover their administrative costs. The corresponding decrease in physician productivity for these medical practices amounts to another significant cost, which will lead to an alarming doctor shortage not too long from now.

The Electronic Health Record Mandate and Decreased Doctor Productivity
EHR has to be implemented to make medical records meaningful and useful; however, the way this implementation is being done today is hampering doctor productivity. Although I have not seen any statistics about the impact of EHRs on physicians' productivity, I estimate that in my own case the mandate dropped my productivity by at least a third. I would have never thought many years ago that my productivity as a physician would be dependent on the speed of my typing to fix the inaccuracies of my voice recognition device. It is difficult for a non-physician to understand this idea that adopting technology would actually decrease productivity, as it is totally different in other industries. EHR is formatted in such a way that doctors spend almost the same amount of time (or sometimes more time) inputting data about a patient as they do seeing the patient!

The old-fashioned method of dictating to an analog device and having a medical transcriptionist type the words out cannot be done here because of the rigid structure of input data, and because only so much of the documentation can be delegated to assistants. There are attempts being made by software developers to make EHRs less demanding at the expense of making the digital record less individualized and more of a series of templates. However, adoption of EHR as it is done today has reduced doctors to data entry clerks for a good portion of their time that should be spent on patient care.

The Effects of the Ever-Changing Diagnosis Classification System
Meanwhile, the complexity of medical coding adds another layer of administrative costs for medical offices. The history of medical codes dates as far back as the 15th century, when physicians in Italy began grouping diseases together in an attempt to better understand their nature and treatment. The 18th century saw the creation of an International List of Causes of Death. That list, originally intended for use in vital statistics, became increasingly utilized by hospitals for indexing medical records. The Great Exhibition of 1851 in London contributed by igniting an interest in comparing statistics internationally, particularly causes of death.[1]

The classification system we use today is a revision of the International Classification of Diseases, better known as ICD. In 2003, the Health Insurance Portability and Accountability Act (HIPAA) of 1996 named ICD-9 as the code set for reporting diagnoses and procedures in electronic administrative transactions. In 2009, the Department of Health and Human Services (HHS) published a regulation requiring the replacement of ICD-9 with ICD-10. Covered entities (health care providers, including physicians, payers, and clearinghouses) are required to comply with this regulation.[2]

Originally set to be implemented in October 2013, ICD-10 was rolled out in October 2015 and is sure to cause further declines in doctors' productivity. ICD-10 created five times the amount of diagnosis codes that ICD-9 has in order to allow for greater specificity. For example, there are four ICD-9 codes relating to hematuria (blood in the urine). With ICD-10, there are over 20 codes that may match hematuria. This massive change will in turn cause an increase in costs for health care providers, both in terms of time and finances. Nachimson Advisors estimated in 2008 the total cost impact of the ICD-10 mandate to be $83,290 per small practice (defined as three doctors and two administrative staff), $285,195 per medium practice (defined as 10 providers, six administrative staff, and one full-time coder), and $2.7 million for a large practice (defined as 100 providers and 64 coding staff, comprised of 10 full-time coders and 54 medical records staff).[3]

The 2014 updated estimates by the same group came up with even more devastating figures: between $56,639 and $226,105 for a small practice, between $213,364 and $824,735 for a medium practice, and between $2,017,151 and $8,018,364 for a large practice.[4] These estimates include the cost of staff education and training, the burden of increased documentation requirements, and the necessary analysis of how the changes affect business processes. While other reports find the costs relating to ICD-10 to be much less exorbitant, there is no question that the transition has created financial and logistical stress for health care providers and continues to decrease physician productivity, which is akin to an increase in health care costs. The coding changes require modifications in practice management software, billing service and clearinghouse vendors, Electronic Health Record vendors, and others. The ICD-10 learning curve is a steep and costly one. Again, this is an administrative cost that is causing solo practices to struggle and eventually die off.

These intricacies have left many health care providers no other alternative than to outsource their billing and coding. As we have discussed, the medical billing and coding industry (the "middleman to the middleman") has enjoyed significant popularity virtually overnight. The Bureau of Labor Statistics (BLS) projects that the increase in employment of medical records and health information technicians (which includes medical billers and coders) from 2012 to 2022 will be 22 percent. This is in comparison to an average growth rate for all occupations that is about 11 percent.[5] This trend is in large part due to the increased demands that ICD-10 will have on health care providers.

A Looming Shortage of Doctors
As we have seen, the administrative costs of medical offices are becoming unbearably large. My prediction is that this will mean there will be a severe shortage of physicians not so far into the future after the full implementation of the Electronic Health Record mandate. To illustrate the frustration felt by many doctors, below are some quotes from physicians around the country who were surveyed in a 2012 study by The Physicians Foundation:

> "There is a shortage of primary care physicians currently. This will be even more acutely felt if too much is asked for them to do as far as regulation is concerned. A majority of them are close to retirement and will just leave if more is expected of them that has little to do with actual patient care. The current trend to increase the regulations will push more of them into retirement."

> "We are inundated with so many rules, seeing a patient is a chore rather than a pleasure. My patient numbers have been cut by 20 percent due to paper regulations and EMR has made it worse. I have been on EMR for eight years and it is not new to me. We focus more on the paperwork than the patient. This is due to regulation and not due to a true desire to establish good relationships."

> "Actually, within one year I will probably close my practice. The local, state, and federal mandates and regulations have overwhelmed my ability to continue as a small businessman. I love being a doctor and I really don't know what I'll do next."

> "I see my future pay reducing substantially with what is

going on in Washington today. If that occurs, I will leave medicine. I do not see, for the years of training required, liability, hours per week... that, given the future loss of physician compensation, there will be enough young, bright individuals interested in medicine."

"As government gets more involved in medicine and threatens cuts, especially Medicare, more and more physicians are saying goodbye to medicine. The result will be poorer health care, by far, a few years from now. Thankfully, I will be out of it, but will have to suffer as a consumer with the consequences of this short-[sighted] reaction."[6]

According to 2012 American Medical Association data, nearly 50 percent of U.S. doctors are over 49 years of age,[7] meaning that they have not used computers for most of their lives and are likely struggling with the increase in typing and documentation related to recent health care mandates. A 2013 survey by Deloitte found that 62 percent of the physicians surveyed anticipate physicians will retire or scale back practice hours based on the way the future of medicine is changing. Six out of ten of the physicians surveyed said that they believe physicians will retire earlier than planned in the next one to three years. The survey found that "this perception is fairly uniform among all physicians, irrespective of age, gender, or medical specialty."[8]

The demand for physicians in the U.S. is increasing, partly because of a large aging population and partly because more Americans are insured and seeking care. It is a real issue that the supply of physicians is not increasing in unison, as you can see in Figure 11.1 on the following page.[9]

IHS, Inc. compiled a report for the Association of American Medical Colleges (AAMC) regarding future physician shortages. The report estimated that in 2025, we will have a shortage of between 46,100 and 90,400 physicians, 12,500 to 31,100 of which will be primary care physicians.[10] In light of our previous discussion on the importance of the PCP's role in the health care system, this shortage will surely have a negative impact on the quality, access, and cost of health care in America.

Figure 11.1
Projected Total Physician Shortfall, 2013-2025

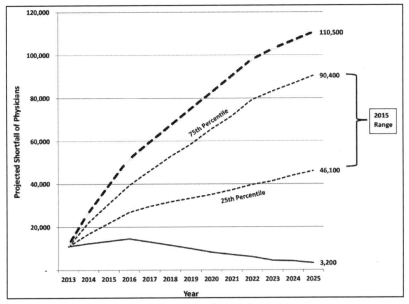

Source: Association of American Medical Colleges

CHAPTER TWELVE
DIRECT-TO-CONSUMER MARKETING BY PHARMACEUTICAL COMPANIES

Recently, and in American culture much more so than in other cultures, we have seen a huge spike in the usage of direct-to-consumer advertising by pharmaceutical companies. I say that this is particularly American because most countries actually do not allow direct-to-consumer pharmaceutical advertising (DTCPA). In fact, the U.S. and New Zealand are the only countries that allow DTCPA that includes product claims.[1] Though DTCPA is regulated by the American federal government's Food and Drug Administration, some criticize that the rules are too lax. DTCPA by drug companies is a rather recent phenomenon which was not made legal until 1985. The advertising took off sharply in 1997 when the FDA relaxed the rules that obligated drug companies to detail side effects of medications. As a result, "advertisers had to include only 'major risks' and provide an 'adequate provision' that would direct viewers elsewhere to access complete 'brief summary' information."[2]

    Heavy advertising by pharmaceutical companies is all over the airwaves and no one can escape it. The magnitude of impact of these direct-to-consumer advertisements through non-medical media outlets like TV, Internet, and magazines is palpable, but difficult to quantify. One study finds that the average American TV viewer watches as many as nine drug ads a day. This comes to about 16 hours a year, which unfortunately far exceeds the amount of time the average individual spends with a primary care physician.[3] Just think, in any given day, how many commercials you see ending with "ask your doctor." We as doctors are on the receiving end of these ads.

Patients often come to me and ask me to write a prescription for something that they had seen on television recently. It is hard to blame them for this, as the skills of the advertisers of Madison Avenue make just about any medical product seem "magical." Therein lies one of the problems: these ads are often quite misleading to the patient. A 2007 study in *The Journal of Health Communication* found that the average direct-to-consumer television commercial devotes more time to benefits than to risks, though this is in violation of the FDA stipulation that an ad must present a "fair balance" of benefits and risks.[4]

Disturbingly, many of these drugs are later rescinded from the market or found out to be misrepresented. Quite often, a product is advertised for years as the panacea to treat a common disorder; just a few years later, if that product is proven harmful, that same exact product advertisement is being used by product liability and personal injury attorneys in their own advertising! We have all seen these types of ads made by lawyers; they play the original pharmaceutical ad and then say something along the lines of, "if you took this medication or used this device and (insert harmful complication or death) happened to you or your loved one, call us and you may be entitled to cash compensation!" A well-known example of this was Vioxx, the infamous non-steroidal anti-inflammatory drug created by Merck, prescribed primarily for the treatment of arthritis. Heavily marketed and widely prescribed from 1999 to 2004, the drug was associated with an increased risk of stroke and heart attack when used at high doses on a long-term basis. It was withdrawn from the market in 2004.[5] Dr. David Graham of the FDA estimated that Vioxx was linked to more than 27,000 heart attacks or sudden cardiac deaths nationwide from the time it came on the market in 1999 through 2003.[6]

Admittedly, it is very difficult to estimate how much direct-to-consumer advertising of pharmaceuticals impacts health care costs. The dramatic increase in the number of prescriptions written in the last 20 years (a far greater increase than in population growth, as discussed in Chapter 5) is abnormal and must be explained. As mentioned briefly, the abnormality is even more puzzling considering that in the last 20 years at least 20 very popular drugs that used to be available only by prescription have become available over-the-counter. The growth in over-the-counter availability of these often-used prescription drugs should actually decrease the number of prescriptions considerably rather than increasing it considerably! The unnatural increase in the number of prescriptions per person in that period coincides with both the surge in direct-to-consumer advertising of drugs and the advent of using physician extenders as a new class of prescribers. These potentially causative relationships would certainly be an interesting area for further research.

SECTION III.
THE DIAGNOSIS: GETTING LESS

With all of these costs in mind, one would hope our health care system produces the very best results. As discussed, however, we are paying far more for health care in the United States, but our performance on metrics of health quality still falls significantly short. This begs the question: where are we going wrong in terms of quality?

We have looked at a variety of metrics in which the U.S. health system fails compared to its counterparts. Life expectancy at birth, as we explored, is the cumulative effect of all aspects of health. An adverse factor that is dramatically bringing down our life expectancy numbers, and making it so that we are too often "getting less," is called iatrogenic disease, or doctor-caused disease. The next two chapters will be devoted to this concept. (The many other health metrics described in Chapter 1 that contribute to U.S. patients "getting less" will not be revisited here.)

A Dual Death
As we explore iatrogenic diseases, we will be highlighting a prime example of the "dual death" concept we have touched upon previously. In exploring the direct and destructive financial impact that medical bills can cause, we could see how bankruptcy represents a sort of "death" of a person's financial being. It is here that we will begin to more clearly see the meaning of the other component of the "dual death" described in the Introduction.

It is quite natural for you to wonder how iatrogenic diseases contribute to American patients "getting less." We will find by the conclusion of this coming chapter that the meaning of "getting less" is very clear, namely getting less of life – both in terms of quantity and health-related quality. We will begin to see – as shocking as it is – the physical, literal death that can be caused directly by health care.

CHAPTER THIRTEEN
IATROGENIC DISEASES: THE THIRD MOST COMMON CAUSE OF DEATH IN THE UNITED STATES

Dying of Health Care Physically

Unless you are in the medical profession, the chances that you knew what the word "iatrogenic" means before picking up this book are slim to none. Over the course of writing this book, I conducted an informal survey among my patients. I asked over 470 of my patients if they knew the meaning of an iatrogenic disease. Only three of them did. Additionally, I asked 26 registered nurses, and only one of them was familiar with the concept. Indeed, most people – even within the health care industry – do not know about the term. However, once you learn more about what it is and the impact it has, you will wonder why this is not a more commonly discussed topic.

The Merriam-Webster dictionary defines iatrogenic as "induced inadvertently by a physician or surgeon or by medical treatment or diagnostic procedures." The Oxford dictionary defines iatrogenic as "of or relating to illness caused by medical examination or treatment." Various other definitions converge on the same meaning: an iatrogenic condition is a disease, injury, or death that a patient experiences as a result of medical or surgical intervention; it is a condition that he or she would not have had otherwise. Essentially, an iatrogenic disease is a case in which the result of medical or surgical intervention is worse than the disease itself.

Iatrogenic comes from a Greek root term *iatros*, meaning

physician, and can be translated to "brought forth by the healer." It is ironic, of course, that a disease would be brought forth by a healer. However, it makes sense that these very unfortunate diseases and deaths would come about at times due to occasional mistakes made by physicians, correct? What we will see, which is quite appalling, is that these diseases occur at a far greater frequency than one might imagine.

For most readers, this concept is very new, and that is okay. As you can see, however, it is so crucial to understand. This is why I have put it at the heart of this book, even in the title itself. As you will see from the examples in this section, iatrogenic disease can alter life dramatically both in terms of quantity and health-related quality.

Real Life Examples
After this rather technical discussion about the definition of iatrogenic diseases, I will now take you into an exploration of two cases I saw early on in my time operating my practice in Florida some 26 years ago. I encountered these two cases within only a few months of one another. Even though I knew the term "iatrogenesis" from my days as a medical student, these two cases profoundly altered my look at "doctor-made diseases" forever. You, as a reader, may not understand their massive impact either, until you consider that it could have been you or your family member in the cases described below.

> 1. *In one absolutely tragic case of an iatrogenic effect, a perfectly healthy nine year-old boy – let us call him Jason – underwent a tonsillectomy (removal of tonsils), which was a common operation at the time. He was not my patient, but his mother was. During anesthesia, Jason sustained brain damage and, after awakening from anesthesia, was unable to talk or move any of his four limbs. He was confined to a wheelchair until he died at the age of 34. His mother, who has been a patient of mine for almost a quarter of a century – let us call her Janet – cared for him daily for more than two decades, from age nine until he died. She nursed him, bathed him, and assisted him in all activities*

that a normally-functioning human being does independently. When he became a teenager, he was a physically large young man compared to his much smaller mother, which only made things more difficult.

Taking care of Jason took an unimaginable toll on Janet's physical and emotional well-being. Jason's life was cut short, and for 25 years he did not have much quality of life either. And the effect did not end with him, as his mother Janet's quality of life was dramatically and tragically diminished as well. Janet is still my patient, even though she moved to a nearby city. She is now 76, and the emotional toll lingers on. She continues to take anti-depressants and has had chronic insomnia for all these years. She was socially withdrawn and isolated during these years as well – understandably so, as she spent most of her time and energy for so long taking care of her son.

2. *The second case is one of a very intelligent, beautiful 31 year-old registered nurse. Let us call her Jessica. I saw Jessica for the first and only time when she was a quadriplegic (paralyzed from the neck down), breathing from a portable oxygen tank. Jessica told me that the quadriplegia was a complication of neck surgery done six years prior for a "pinched nerve."*

Jessica moved to another state after that visit, so I do not have much more information about her life since then. Normally a disability like Jessica's has a definite effect of shortening life expectancy, because the physical dysfunction leads to a myriad of other complications that may cut life short (like in the case of Jason, who died at 34 – less than half of his life expectancy at birth). The main takeaway here is that a neck surgery, which was not due to cancer, caused a young woman to not be able to move her four limbs for the rest of her life. The consequence of the pinched nerve itself would have been nowhere near as devastating in terms of quality or quantity of life. As in Jason's case, the medical intervention made things exponentially worse, and that is a huge understatement.

Both Jason's and Jessica's cases are examples of the

complications of surgery and anesthesia, regardless of where their respective surgeries fit on the spectrum of necessary to unnecessary (which will be discussed in the next chapter). In both cases, life was decreased in both quantity and quality by a doctor's intervention.

These potential complications of surgery and anesthesia are generally considered acceptable. Of course, it is unreasonable to expect that surgeries and anesthesia are risk-free. In fact, whether you are the president of a country, a king, the Pope, or an average citizen, you sign an informed consent form before surgery and anesthesia indicating that you understand that death is one of the potential complications. What I am advocating, however, is that the risk of having surgery and anesthesia be carefully weighed against the potential benefit of the surgery or invasive procedure itself. Surgery for a perforated bowel, for example, is absolutely worth the risk, because it is a life-saving surgery. Death is near-certain without it. But this is not the case for other surgeries in which the benefit is questionable.

Iatrogenic Diseases: The Statistics

Tragically, the examples I have shared are more common than any of us may have imagined. Let us shed some light on the startling magnitude of this issue. In her commentary in *The Journal of the American Medical Association*, Dr. Barbara Starfield of Johns Hopkins University, citing three previous studies, estimated the number of American deaths due to iatrogenic causes to be 225,000 per year. In other words, about 225,000 American deaths per year are actually *caused* by medical care. If it were classified as such, this would make iatrogenic causes the third most common cause of death in the United States, after heart disease and cancer.[1]

To make matters worse, as Dr. Starfield points out, these numbers may actually be on the lower end of comparable estimations. Other estimations arrive at a number of deaths between 230,000 and 284,000. On the lower end, in an article published in *The International Journal of Epidemiology*, Dr. John Bunker estimated between 75,000 and 150,000 iatrogenic deaths in the U.S. annually, including those that result from medical error.[2] And these figures only consider iatrogenic causes of death; they do not include disability or discomfort that have iatrogenic causes.

In 1999, the U.S. Institute of Medicine's (IOM) Committee on Quality of Health Care in America published a landmark report entitled "To Err Is Human: Building a Safer Health System." In it, the results of two studies were extrapolated to estimate that between 44,000 and 98,000 deaths occurred annually in the U.S. due to medical errors in hospitals. Even when using the lower end of this estimate, the report cited that this would make hospital medical errors the 8th leading cause of death in the U.S., claiming more lives annually than breast cancer, AIDS, or motor vehicle accidents.[3] These estimations appear to be conservative as they relate to our topic of conversation, considering iatrogenic effects can and do occur outside of hospitals, and medical errors are not the only source of iatrogenesis.

Estimates of iatrogenic effects vary widely. Compiling this type of data is very difficult, partly because reporting of cases of this kind, for obvious reasons, is incomplete and inaccurate. In the absence of current and reliable data, we cannot put an accurate figure to the incidence of iatrogenic diseases in America. But we can gather from the above estimations that iatrogenic effects are not rare and that the American medical system itself is a significant cause of death and injury in the U.S. Tragically, too many of us are dying... dying of health care.

Simple Mathematical Conclusions: Paying More and Getting Less Quantity and Health-related Quality of Life

In reading the summary of what iatrogenic diseases are and how prevalent they are in America, three clear conclusions shine through in my mind:

1. When tens of thousands die every year in the U.S. due to iatrogenic causes, many will be young people, or at least people who are not near the end of their natural lives. This will then be responsible for dragging down the mathematical average of life expectancy, which, as we

know, is an area in which the United States ranks on the low end when compared with other developed countries. Iatrogenic deaths are thus a driver of this lower life expectancy. In other words, iatrogenesis contributes to a decrease in life quantity.

2. If tens of thousands of people die from iatrogenic diseases every year, you can probably safely assume that at least double this number are injured or disabled because of the same types of causes that lead to iatrogenic deaths. Remember that cases like Jason's and Jessica's – although the medical intervention ultimately led to severely shortened and more difficult lives – are not officially considered iatrogenic deaths. Their cases and similar ones are considered iatrogenic injuries or disabilities. We saw from those examples just how terribly those injuries or disabilities can affect a person's life. In other words, iatrogenesis contributes to a decrease in health-related quality of life.

3. The iatrogenic diseases, whether they end in death or disability, cost a good deal of money. Thus, they affect both sides of the "paying more to get less" paradox. The crux of this book – the dual financial and physical death of the American patient at the hands of the system – is best illustrated here.

I will end this chapter with a kinder note about our profession. The significant increase in life expectancy in the last one hundred years in the U.S. and around the world is mostly a function of modern medicine and surgery, especially progress within the areas of vaccinations and antibiotics. We do not claim in the medical profession that we have a "silver bullet" for every disease, but the sacred trust patients put in us to do our best with what we know will always be honored under any circumstance. It is our solemn oath. Unfortunately for American doctors, however, it is our current health care delivery system that creates an environment leading to suboptimal results in nearly all metrics of health quality when compared across similar nations.

CHAPTER FOURTEEN
DISSECTING IATROGENIC DISEASES

Joan Rivers, the American actress, comedian, and television host, went to a clinic for a laryngoscopy (a procedure to visualize the voice box) and an upper gastrointestinal endoscopy (a procedure to visualize the upper digestive tract) and died as a result of complications during a procedure in which several errors were made. There are thousands of Americans who die every year in similar fashions. Unfortunately, not many hear about these thousands and thousands of silent deaths because the victims may not be as famous or influential as someone like Joan Rivers. The immense pain inflicted on these people's families, however, is something that everyone should know about and work to fix. It is a terrible injustice.

By the Way, More Costs!
In the introduction to Section II, we briefly noted that one major cost was going to come up in this section: the cost of iatrogenic diseases. Indeed, iatrogenic diseases are not just a harrowing example of American patients "getting less" in terms of medical treatment, but also a striking example of a major cost to the American health care system. In this way, it is a fascinating case in how paying more and getting less are so inextricably tied together.

There are a variety of sub-classifications within the larger topic of "iatrogenic effects." We will explore a few of these below.

Related to Medications
The most common iatrogenic effects seem to be drug-related. As

we touched on before, compiling accurate data about iatrogenic diseases and deaths is impossible because of poor reporting due to fear of liability. There is also a more important reason specifically connected to drug-related effects: most drug-related deaths are likely to occur in a non-hospital setting, so it is difficult for the family or the family physician to know the cause of death. Thus, it will be presumed to be from a natural cause like a heart attack. For these reasons, estimates are the only thing we have to judge the magnitude of the problem. A study published in *The Journal of the American Medical Association* in 1998 estimated that, in 1994, adverse drug reactions were responsible for ending 106,000 lives in the U.S., making these reactions between the fourth and sixth leading cause of death.[1]

Many of the non-fatal effects may not be apparent either to the patient or the doctor until irreversible damage has already occurred. So, studies measuring the magnitude of the problem are bound to be conservative. A study conducted in an internal medicine department found that 22.9 percent of patients studied experienced an iatrogenic event. Most of the iatrogenic events in the series – nearly 60 percent – were drug-related, followed by those resulting from technical procedures. Over 60 percent of the drug-related iatrogenic illnesses were due to side effects or adverse drug reactions (ADRs), 20 percent to inappropriate dosing, and 10 percent to drug interactions.[2] The more medications that are being taken, the greater the risk of adverse effects. As discussed in Chapter 5, polypharmacy exponentially increases the chances of having an adverse reaction that causes harm or death. This is yet another example of paying more to get less.

There is no doubt that introductions of several classes of medicines have improved patients' quantities and qualities of life. Just one of these classes is proton pump inhibitors (PPIs), which are medications that suppress acid secretion and are used in the treatment of stomach ulcers. The advent of the first member of this class was in the early 1990s and it made the treatment of stomach ulcers simpler. In fact, elective (non-emergency) surgery as treatment for chronic ulcers was commonplace before the advent of this class of drugs, but since the introduction of PPIs, surgery as treatment has all but vanished. An emergency surgery for perforation of the ulcer, which is life threatening, was also common; young doctors do not see these any more thanks to PPIs.

However, this does not change the fact that many drugs are ineffective and harmful. Much of this is well-illustrated by a 2007 book called *Overtreated: Why Too Much Medicine Makes Us Sicker and Poorer*, written by award-winning journalist Shannon Brownlee. In this book, Brownlee describes in great detail this glaring example of paying more to get less. As suggested by the book title, which may seem to be counterintuitive to the average reader, the tragic and sad truth is that the increase in drugs has actually hurt our nation's citizens both physically and financially. Overtreatment, as I have seen in nearly four decades of practicing medicine, can indeed make a patient sicker or cause him or her to die poor.

Related to Hospital Stays

Complications and deaths considered in this section are directly related to the hospital stay and are not related to the reason the patient was hospitalized. These iatrogenic diseases related to hospital stays include hospital-acquired infections (nosocomial infections), blood clots, bedsores, and medication errors, among others. In a 2010 report by the Health and Human Services Office of the Inspector General (OIG) team, it was concluded that the rate of harm among hospitalized Medicare patients was 27 percent. Half of these patients experienced one or more adverse events that resulted in a prolonged hospital stay, permanent harm, a life-sustaining intervention, or death, and almost half of all events identified in the OIG report were considered preventable.[3] Another article published in 2007 estimated that 1.7 million health care-associated infections (HAIs) occurred in U.S. hospitals in 2002 and were associated with approximately 99,000 deaths.[4] Some studies have found that anywhere from 3.7 to 17 percent of all patients admitted to a hospital experience an iatrogenic effect of some kind.[5] A 1997 study conducted at two prestigious teaching hospitals found that about two out of every 100 admissions experienced a preventable adverse drug event, resulting in a cost of $2.8 million annually for a 700-bed teaching hospital.[6] Other than adverse drug effects, many iatrogenic effects occurring in hospitals have to do with technical, diagnostic, and therapeutic procedures and their complications. The technical causes of iatrogenic effects in the previously referenced internal medicine department study were mainly associated with catheterization, with surgery a distant second (see Figure 14.1 below).[7]

**Figure 14.1
Types of Iatrogenic Disease
Due to Technical Causes in an Internal Medicine Department**

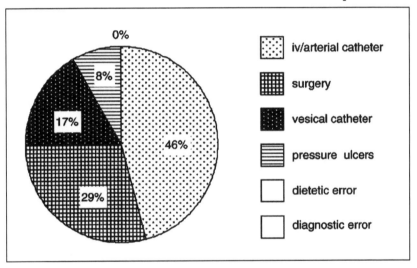

Source: European Journal of Internal Medicine

A nosocomial infection is by definition a hospital-acquired infection. According to an article by Dr. William Jarvis, about two million nosocomial infections occur in the U.S. per year.[8] Another source indicates that the incidence of nosocomial infections in hospitalized patients in internal medicine wards can be as high as 2.6 percent.[9] Most of these incidents are associated with bloodstream infections, pneumonia, surgical site infections, and urinary tract infections (UTIs). Because antibiotics are prevalent in the hospital environment, the organisms causing these infections frequently develop antibiotic resistance and thus the infections are difficult to treat. Examples of such organisms are Methicillin-Resistant Staphylococcus Aureus (MRSA) and Clostridium difficile (C-dif). Nosocomial infections require treatment and prolonged stays in the hospital, which creates an added economic burden. As we seek to reduce the incidence of nosocomial infections, we will be reducing the costs associated with treating these cases. Controlling infection is cost-effective as well as life-preserving.

Related to Unnecessary Surgeries, Procedures, and Anesthesia
The thought of having unnecessary surgery is disturbing, but the thought of dying during an unnecessary surgery is unspeakable. Before you start pointing an accusatory finger at surgeons, let us discuss how this may happen in the first place.

What is considered a necessary or unnecessary surgery is extremely subjective. There is not a binary answer that the patient can expect to hear from his or her surgeon. Necessary versus unnecessary surgery is not black and white. Rather, it is more of a spectrum, ranging from life-saving and strongly-indicated, to marginally-beneficial and not strongly-indicated, to outright unnecessary. Of course, cosmetic surgery is in a different category altogether, since the patient is the only one who decides whether surgery is "necessary" or not.

To illustrate this: surgery for a perforated gut is absolutely necessary and is a life-saving surgery. However, a ventral hernia (a relatively common hernia occurring in the upper abdomen, especially in men), except in extreme cases, poses no risk, so surgery is unnecessary. There are numerous examples that lie in between these, filling the spectrum. Where the surgeon's answer falls within the spectrum differs according to the "Four Dimensions" discussed previously. It is also unrealistic to expect that other motives do not influence a surgeon's assessment of the surgery being necessary or unnecessary when it falls in the "grey" area.

In a 1989 article entitled "Unnecessary Surgery," Dr. Lucian Leape defined unnecessary surgery, for the purpose of his study, as such: "[A surgery that] does not do what it purports to do, or at the most, carries benefits so small that they are outweighed by the costs in terms of risks, morbidity, disability, and pain. The patient is not better off."[10]

One must consider that surgery and anesthesia carry an inherent risk, at times being fatal. The amount of risk that is tolerable is dependent on how much added benefit is possible. By this token, no amount of risk is tolerable if there is no possibility of significant benefit. With this in mind, an unnecessary surgery is essentially a surgery that puts the patient at risk without promise of any added benefit when compared to other treatment options.

As we mentioned previously, unnecessary surgeries and procedures are a significant driver of health care costs. One study found that between 13 and 32 percent of surgeries were unnecessary, and some concluded that when it comes to very controversial surgeries, as many as 30 percent are unnecessary.[11]

Additionally, a *USA Today* study found that unnecessary surgeries might account for 10 to 20 percent of all operations in some specialties. Cardiac procedures, such as stents and angioplasties, as well as spinal surgery, knee replacements, and hysterectomies, are among the surgical procedures performed more often than needed, according to a review of in-depth studies and data generated by both government and academic sources.[12]

Furthermore, a 2011 study published in *The Journal of the American Medical Association* looked at nearly 112,000 patients who had an implantable cardioverter-defibrillator (ICD), a pacemaker-like device that corrects heartbeat irregularities. Among them, 22.5 percent did not meet the evidence-based criteria for implantation, and there was one excess complication for every 121 non-evidence-based ICD implantations.[13]

And similarly, a 2011 study published in *Surgical Neurology International* evaluated 274 patients over the course of one year that presented with back and/or neck pain and had been scheduled for spinal operations by an outside surgeon. One neurosurgeon reevaluated all these patients and found that almost 17 percent of these cases were scheduled for "unnecessary surgery," meaning their neurological and radiographic findings were not abnormal.[14]

There are a few main reasons that these unnecessary procedures occur, and those reasons are similar to the ones we mentioned previously in reference to unnecessary testing. For one, the doctor's lack of awareness about recent medical advances may lead to unnecessary surgery or procedures. Practicing evidence-based medicine is of utmost importance. If the doctor is unaware of the most recent studies and data, he or she may not be making the correct recommendation. A surgical procedure may have the same outcome as a nonsurgical treatment, but the doctor may unwisely determine that surgery is the best option for a patient. Greed, which cannot be honestly or realistically ruled out, also plays into this. This is particularly the case when the need for surgery falls in the grey area of the spectrum between necessary and unnecessary, and the subjective opinion of the surgeon is the determining factor. As we discussed previously, the fee-for-service nature of American health care essentially rewards those providers who conduct more surgeries, procedures, and tests.

Some ways of combatting this problem of unnecessary surgery include:

1. Creating a way to disseminate current research, recent trends, and general consensus of effectiveness of surgical treatments or invasive procedures to doctors.

2. Using evidence based medicine (EBM). According to Dr. David Sackett, the definition of EBM is the "integration of the best research evidence with clinical expertise and patient values to make clinical decisions."[15]

3. Using a second opinion. In the grey areas where the indication for surgery is not clear-cut, the "necessity" of the procedure is in the eye of the beholder, or surgeon in this case. Essentially, the opinion is a function of the "Four Dimensions" aforementioned in the "making of a doctor."

4. Standardizing the decision-making process, as I will

advocate later in the book. In determining whether a surgery or procedure is "necessary" or "unnecessary," there will always be an element of subjectivity. But a standardization method will definitely help to reduce that subjectivity. It is worth noting here (and will be discussed later on) that this can only be implemented under a single-payer system with the authority to enforce this standard.

Killing Two Birds with One Stone
The take-home message here is that iatrogenic effects occur at an alarmingly high rate, and steps need to be taken to reduce this rate. Many of the studies cited in this chapter found that iatrogenic effects are often preventable and avoidable.

It is interesting that identifying the causes of iatrogenic diseases and subsequently preventing them could actually decrease the cost of health care while simultaneously increasing the quality of care. It is a case of "killing two birds with one stone," and one that can have a massive impact on our health care system.

The idea that health care can hurt or disable patients both financially and physically is largely what motivated this long-time primary care physician to write this book. It is an egregious injustice. Indeed, the factors that drive up our health care costs are some of the same factors that contribute to our decreased quality and quantity of life. As we will see in the upcoming "treatment" section of the book, preventing sickness and death from iatrogenic diseases is also part of the remedy to treat the high cost of health care.

SECTION IV.
PREPARING FOR THE PRESCRIPTION

As a doctor, it is not always a good idea to jump straight from the diagnosis to the prescription for the treatment. This is especially true if there is crucial context to be laid out, or if it will be a sensitive or difficult conversation. Similarly, in our analysis of the American health care system, there are a couple of topics we should engage with before we hear the treatment so that we can better understand and receive it. These topics – the economics of health care and journalistic sensationalism/political demagoguery – are what we will focus on in this pre-treatment discussion.

CHAPTER FIFTEEN
FROM MACROECONOMICS TO HEALTH CARE ECONOMICS: WHY OUR PATH IS UNSUSTAINABLE

Medicine and economics have something crucial in common. Just as we saw that medicine is an inexact science, so too is economics. This means that practitioners in each field can and do have different opinions when presented with the same exact data. We have already discussed the differences of opinion within medicine. Now, let us explore economics in general, and then specifically explore how this relates to the economics of health care. My intent is not to weary you with a lot of technical discussion on economics. However, to understand the solution to health care problems, one must understand the larger economic environment of which health care economics is a part. Even if you know nothing about economics, I hope you will find this chapter revealing and interesting.

Consumption, Production, and Standard of Living
The gross domestic product (GDP) is the aggregate total of a nation's output of goods and services. Think of the GDP as the size of the economy. The act of providing services (including health care) constitutes a large percentage of America's GDP. Health care expenditure is considered "consumption." Even though you need a healthy workforce to produce goods, health care falls into the service sector of the economy rather than the goods-producing sector. Now, when you cut health care expenditures, you decrease economic activity in the short run. However, this frees up capital that can be redirected and used for "production" – the

development of innovative new services and products.

A nation's standard of living is the level of wealth available to people in that nation. Standard of living improves via production, not via consumption. If part of the consumption is paid for by debt, this means that it will be paid later on from future consumption (this is a situation of "short-term gain versus long-term pain"). Unless production and productivity increase far beyond the money borrowed for consumption, the future standard of living will decrease. "Paying the piper" will have to happen sooner or later. This is easy-to-understand economics, and we should keep this in mind throughout our discussion about health care economics. Simply consuming more health care resources is not a solution to our ailing system, especially when said consumption is not producing better health care results.

Differing Opinions in Economics, Differing Opinions in Medicine
As we have said, practitioners in economics and in medicine can disagree about quite a lot of things. Many economists have different opinions on this topic of production and consumption and on a wide range of other topics.

To illustrate the diversity of perspectives in economics, let us consider some of the most well-known economists and their diverging views. Let us start with Keynesian economics. There was a British economist in the Depression era of the 1930s by the name John Maynard Keynes who became popular worldwide through advocating the idea that governments can stimulate economies in bad times by running a budget deficit. They can pay back borrowed money when they eventually run a surplus during economic recovery by increasing tax receipts. Modern-day followers of Keynes, often called Keynesian economists, often betray him by adhering to only the first part of his suggestion that governments can keep borrowing money and spending it. When governments run out of lenders, they resort to their central banks to print money (the Federal Reserve is America's central bank). The modern-day version of money printing is called quantitative easing, which functions the same as old-fashioned printing of money. This increasing of the monetary supply then decreases the value of existing currency, reducing its purchasing power. This process is called inflation. In the eyes of Keynesians, consumption is the key to prosperity, regardless of where the money for consumption comes from. This includes the act of borrowing that money for consumption, whether the borrowing is done by individuals, corporations, or the government itself.

Perhaps the most famous Keynesian economist today is Nobel Prize winner and *New York Times* columnist Paul Krugman. Krugman once suggested that a simulated alien invasion would cure unemployment by spurring economic activity to fend off that invasion. We would have to build, presumably, defenses and underground cities, so people would be employed to accomplish these things. Of course, he is right in that the economy would boom in the short run and that unemployment would be cured temporarily. Indeed, this would even create a severe shortage of labor! What Paul Krugman failed to mention, however, is that money spent on these massive defense projects is borrowed money. Borrowed money needs to be paid later. Also, these underground cities are inert, non-productive projects; they do not add any new or improved services or goods to society. The economic "pain" will come later. Even if the projects are financed indirectly by the Federal Reserve creating money, the "piper" will be paid later by hyperinflation. Remember, short-term gain leads to long-term pain.

This "simulated alien invasion curing unemployment" idea can be likened to the idea of deliberately tearing down a sizable percentage of government buildings and schools in order to rebuild them. Again, this will spur economic activity through a building boom that will in turn stimulate other kinds of economic activity. With certainty, there will be no unemployed people left in the short term, but the misery comes when paying later. At least in this example, there is use for the rebuilt government buildings and schools (but, of course, there are the lost assets of the purposefully torn down ones), unlike the underground cities in the simulated alien invasion, which would be useless economically. Ultimately, my key message is that production is what matters in the long run, not simply consumption, and that this production is what allows debts to be paid back.

Many economists disagree with Krugman and Keynes. Differences in opinion among economists are perhaps even more divergent than those among medical practitioners. Indeed, there are different schools of economic thought that differ sometimes dramatically from Keynesianism. Some examples are:

1. Supply Side Economics. Economist Arthur Laffer, the creator of the well-known "Laffer Curve," famously champions this school of thought. This school's thinkers were the architects of "Reaganomics" during Ronald Reagan's presidency. They argue that lowering the tax rate spurs economic growth and in turn causes an increase in tax revenue. This school of thought is almost the opposite of Keynesianism.

2. Monetarism. Economists Milton Friedman (who also won a Nobel Prize) and Anna Schwartz were the most popular advocates of this school. It believes that the central bank (in our case the Federal Reserve) can control economic output through controlling money supply.

3. Austrian School of Economics. Austrian economist Ludwig von Mises led a branch of this school of economic thought. It believes that economies go through natural cycles, and government should not intervene to influence these cycles. It also believes that sound monetary policy of a government's central bank means making its paper money backed by gold. This school of economic thought is central to the economic convictions of the former presidential candidate and congressman Dr. Ron Paul. This school disagrees with almost every principle for which Keynesianism stands.

As you see in these examples, even a Nobel Prize winner can have an opinion with which many – including myself (and I am a non-economist, so this may seem on the surface as a blasphemous act) and different Nobel Prize winners in the same exact field – differ. Doctors are not alone in their differences of opinion; not even a Nobel Prize winner is likely able to settle the differences of opinion in medicine or in economics!

I hope this extended discussion of differing opinions in economics shows you one important thing: ideas can diverge dramatically even among intelligent people and experts in the same field. With regard to the health care discussion, I hope that this will encourage you to be an independent thinker as we go through the "treatment" portion of this book. Ultimately, I hope that you will consider the potential solutions pragmatically, leaving behind any beliefs advanced by political ideologues or self-proclaimed pundits who see health care problems from a narrow prism.

Getting Sick or "Dying" Financially Because of Health Care
All of this talk about economics and the importance of production leads us to the economic conundrum caused by the American health care system. The financial health effects occur on three levels:

> *Individuals*: On the individual level, we have seen how high health care costs affect Americans: the most common cause of bankruptcy in the U.S. is medical bills. Struggling individuals and families face a "financial death" in the case of bankruptcy, forcing them to start a new financial life.

> *Corporations*: What happens at the corporate level? Corporations live and die by profits. The profits are a function of cost efficiency. If a global company is based in the United States (for example, General Motors) and spends a lot more on the health care of its employees than another competing global company based in another country (for example, Toyota in Japan), there is a competitive

disadvantage. These companies that must pay more for health care are incentivized to move their operations or they may "die" financially and cease to exist due to their inability to compete in the global marketplace.

The Government: Finally, there is the government level. Government health care costs constitute part of America's yearly budget deficit, which, with its cumulative effect, becomes our national debt. And our national debt is now nearly $19 trillion. In thinking about debt, it helps to consider that governments and individuals are somewhat alike. When the ratio of debt compared to income reaches a certain level that is beyond a person's ability to service it, we run into issues that I call financial "death." In the long run, spending cannot exceed earning on a continuous basis. The same is true for governments. Unlike individuals or corporations, governments do not die financially – they have options that often come at a very high cost to their citizens' standard of living.

When we more deeply explore the case of governments (and the U.S. government in particular), though, it gets a bit more complex. Most of the components that constitute the future liability of the U.S. government, like Social Security for instance, are easily calculable (there is a specific formula for Social Security, actually). Health care expenditures (Medicare and Medicaid), however, are impossible to gauge into the future. They comprise somewhat of a black hole. In fact, Laurence Kotlikoff, an economics professor at Boston University, estimates the total government indebtedness including all future unfunded liabilities, or "fiscal gap," is actually more than 12 times the current GDP. Kotlikoff estimated that this fiscal gap was as high as $210 trillion (that is $210,000,000,000,000) in 2013, while the GDP was nearly $17 trillion.[1] That comes to about $656,000 per person. After reading that, you may either disbelieve the number and dismiss the whole book as fiction, or you may believe it and become scared. In fact, several other experts have come to generally the same conclusion, albeit at a lower figure. Regardless of the exact figure, the reality of the situation is frightening. This incomprehensibly high number is largely due to the current liability of health care mandates and the unpredictable and impossible-to-gauge size of future health expenditures. As we have explored, health care costs already account for about 17 percent of our GDP. In the coming years, as the Congressional Budget Office's 2014 annual budget outlook states, without action the deficit will grow noticeably larger due to the rising health care costs we have discussed, combined with our aging population and expanding federal subsidies for health insurance.[2]

So, the financial outlook is grim, and health care costs are a huge part of the problem. What are the consequences?

Unlike individuals, when a government cannot service its debt, it cannot obtain bankruptcy protection from court. When governments have excessive debt burden (debt compared to the size of the economy, or debt-to-GDP ratio), the best scenario is that the country's rate of increase in economic growth outpaces the rate by which the debt-to-GDP ratio increases. The problem occurs when the debt-to-GDP ratio reaches a certain level at which it ceases to enhance economic growth, but instead hampers it. In a 2010 analysis of 44 industrialized and developing economies over two centuries, economists Carmen Reinhart and Kenneth Rogoff determined that level, or "threshold," of public debt to be 90 percent of GDP. (Today, the U.S. debt-to-GDP ratio is over 100 percent). Reinhart and Rogoff found that "across both advanced countries and emerging markets, high debt/GDP levels (90 percent and above) are associated with notably lower growth outcomes."[3] When debt levels begin to adversely affect growth to a point at which the debt-to-GDP ratio increases faster than growth, it makes the aforementioned favorable outcome a mathematical impossibility. In that case, only two options remain. One is to default on the debt and thus increase interest rates, as lenders to the government will consider the government to be a credit risk. That marked rise in interest rate will create a depression. The other option is to inflate the debt away through the central bank creating money (quantitative easing). Both options are extremely painful and will dramatically decrease the standard of living of citizens. The first option does so through decreased economic activity or depression and the second option does so through hyperinflation that dramatically decreases the purchasing power of the rapidly depreciating currency.

Conclusions from the Economics Discussion
From this discussion on economics, we should feel empowered to think independently and examine the facts pragmatically, for even Nobel Prize winners do not have a monopoly on the truth. We can conclude that:

1. There is no such thing as the proverbial "free lunch" in economics. Short-term gain is often followed by much more severe long-term pain.

2. Health care resources are finite, like everything else. If you spend more on one thing, it comes from what could be spent on another.

3. Current health care spending cannot be sustained or afforded. The health care expenditure path the United States is currently on will certainly lead to extremely painful consequences unless something is done. Ironically, increasing health care expenditures does NOT make us healthier, as we have seen from various statistics and examples. Indeed, we have explored numerous cases throughout this book of instances in which spending more on health care actually leads to worse results.

So, as we proceed into the treatment portion of this book, we must keep in mind the importance of thinking independently and the urgent need to control health care costs while increasing quality of care. We must ensure that financial sickness and death at all levels is avoided, and we must do so by decreasing physical sickness and death as well. Needless to say, there is much work to be done. However, as we will see, many of the solutions described here help to avert both types of death concurrently.

CHAPTER SIXTEEN
GETTING IMMUNIZED AGAINST JOURNALISTIC SENSATIONALISM AND POLITICAL DEMAGOGUERY

There is one more thing that I believe is critical in preparing for the treatment: learning how to discern what is journalistic sensationalism and political demagoguery, and what is truth. The goal is for you to be immunized against sensationalism and demagoguery so that once you hear the half-truth arguments that journalists and politicians often use in their headlines and speeches, you will see through them.

Whenever the issue of reforming the American health care system comes up, you will undoubtedly hear a number of comments and headlines that are meant to arouse emotions and create snap opinions. They are comments like a politician saying "government-run health care will have the same level of efficiency as the post office." These misleading and pseudo-logical statements convey a convincing message to someone who does not look further into the conversation.

In the past few years, I have had discussions comparing public and private health care systems with individuals who knew that I had experience in the public health system of the U.K. These individuals would cite their criticism of the public system based on a single headline. For instance, "I heard this (from someone)" or "I read this (somewhere)," without any details given. They would usually cite Canada, the U.K., and Australia in these headlines. Obviously, these individuals based their opinions on a journalist's writing.

I have included the following illustrations as examples of possible headlines that could appear in an American newspaper or a broadcast, creating a potential "source" of the aforementioned individuals' opinions.

1. "An Australian woman was denied hip replacement surgery for severe osteoarthritis."

2. "A Canadian man crossed the border to get treatment at a Mayo Clinic in the U.S., because he could not have had the same treatment in Canada's public health system."

3. "A British woman died while waiting six months to have surgery."

These storylines are meant to scare the American public; they are examples of journalistic sensationalism. Stopping at these statements alone – as many people do – will certainly stir emotions and inflame passion.

However, we now know that these countries – Australia, Canada, and Britain – tend to perform better in health care metrics than the U.S. and pay far less per person in health care expenditures. I personally practiced in the United Kingdom for a little more than six years in the late 1970s and early 1980s, so I have first-hand experience with the system. I found my health care at the time to be not only readily accessible but also of the highest quality (and I paid very little to the government from my payroll for this). It is certain that the British public health system is not perfect either; it has its pitfalls. However, taken collectively, the problems in the British system, in my experience, are nothing compared to the enormous problems of the U.S. system. So, let us dig deeper into these provocative headlines to find out what is going on. Here we will consider what could have been the real story behind these misleading headlines:

1. The Australian woman is 95 years old, most likely a patient

who has dementia due to Alzheimer's disease in addition to her hip osteoarthritis. She has had multiple strokes. Additionally, let us consider a hypothetical for the sake of discussion: her great grandchild was born with a polycystic kidney, which will kill the child during early life unless he has a kidney transplant. The child will be able to get this transplant as soon as a kidney donor is found. There is only enough money to treat one of the two members of the family, as both operations are incredibly expensive. (As we will see in Chapter 18, this hypothetical situation is an appropriate microcosm of the decisions that must be made with our finite health resources at a national level).

2. This Canadian man who sought treatment in the U.S. is most likely very wealthy. He has several hundred million dollars, and – needless to say – a great deal of disposable income. He, sadly, has a destroyed heart and lungs due to many years of smoking. He is seeking an experimental treatment of a heart-lung transplant that costs probably one million dollars, or perhaps even more health care resources, and is only available in the U.S. Additionally, the treatment, if successful, is only likely to prolong his life for a few months at best.

3. The British woman most likely died of another disease that had nothing to do with the surgery for which she was waiting.

After reading these contexts, you come away with a dramatically different perspective on each situation, right? The response of the average person who stays in the conversation long enough to hear the second half of these three stories will be tempered significantly, regardless of his or her political beliefs or convictions. However, sensationalism and demagoguery will choose the first set of headlines and limit discussion of the context. It would do a world of good if we all kept this in mind as we discuss the potential remedies for our health care system both in this book and in all future conversations.

The truth, in fact, is that the United States is the only Western developed country without universal health care. The U.S. remains an outlier. Given our system's dismal results and untenable costs, we must be open to honestly and genuinely grapple with potential solutions. We must consider these ideas by their merit and not merely by the often ideologically-driven headlines we see or hear.

SECTION V.
PRESCRIBING THE TREATMENT

At long last, we are ready for the prescription! With our rather comprehensive diagnosis in mind, we can now look to the potential solutions for this ailing American health care system. We have a solid understanding of the many, often interconnected problems that are causing our health care to cost so much more than that of any other place in the world while providing us limited quality. We also have a working understanding of economics from a health care perspective, as well as an awareness of how the media often misleads the public into feeling negatively about certain policy proposals and ideas.

I am privileged to have a unique perspective from which to offer my treatment suggestions. Firstly, I am a member of the medical profession, and no health care economist or administrator can fully understand the inner workings of the medical profession more so than a member of that profession. Secondly, I am a practicing primary care physician, and have been for almost 40 years. Unlike specialists, practicing PCPs are in the center of health care and have a panoramic view of the system as a whole, rather than just a sector of it. Thirdly, I have worked in the U.K., within a mostly public health care system in which there is no fee-for-service method of payment, so I understand the potential interrelationship between money and health care from a different standpoint. Lastly, I understand economics enough to make the connection between macroeconomics and health care economics, which, as you will see, is a crucial connection.

With all of this, we can commence the prescription stage.

CHAPTER SEVENTEEN
CREATE A SINGLE-PAYER WITH AUTHORITY

Any discussion about health care reform is always politically charged. America's health care problems as they stand now are a "cancer" that threatens our socioeconomic well-being. It is treatable at the moment, but will prove to be fatal if treatment is delayed. So, we need to be open-minded about the potential treatment options. Trust me: the taste of the medicine or the thought of having the surgery that will cure you is often unpleasant. I am certainly an independent thinker and do not subscribe to ideological dogmas of the conservative right or liberal left. I would encourage you all to look at this issue from the same unbiased standpoint, which is why I sought to immunize you against journalistic sensationalism and political demagoguery in the preceding chapter.

That said, to tackle the problems we have discussed, there must be a single powerful entity that can administer health care and make uniform decisions for the sake of the patients' well-being: a "single-payer." I urge you to please leave behind any preconceived notion you may have on the topic and think pragmatically. All other industrialized Western nations have come to similar conclusions and adopted public health.

Too Good to Be True?
There are not many times in life that you are presented with a multifaceted, complex problem like health care and are able to find a "silver bullet" that solves most, if not all, aspects of the problem in one simple shot. It sounds too good to be true but – in this case

– it is not!

For those who are wary of greater government involvement, do not worry. The "single-payer" does not have to be the government. It could be a non-profit health insurer like Blue Cross Blue Shield, a non-profit organization like Kaiser Permanente (which often pioneers health care cost containment initiatives), a health care cooperative, or a yet-to-be-thought-of, innovative entity if the government-run system strikes fear in the hearts of many citizens. However, I would ask you to at least consider the government as a candidate for that single-payer role. It has the authority and, in running both Medicare and Medicaid, relevant experience. Administratively, the single-payer would likely work best as the government. Just think about it and do not reject it out of hand.

The Major Advantages of a Single-Payer
The advantage of this structure, regardless of who the single-payer organization may be, is that it will provide one entity with the authority to reduce almost all of the waste in the system. That single-payer will have the power to:

1. Eliminate the waste surrounding administrative costs of insurers and billing companies. The existing infrastructure of health insurance administration can be used but, as you would expect, much less capacity would be needed.

2. Negotiate prices with pharmaceutical companies and device manufacturers, thus bringing down prices to be more in line with the far cheaper prices these companies are selling their products for overseas. This negotiating power can be used to negotiate expensive technology items like MRI scanners, robotic surgery tools, and the like. These big-ticket items are some of the most important factors driving expensive hospital charges, which make up a significant portion of health care expenditure. Perhaps the single-payer can purchase these big-ticket items and lease them to hospitals,

but of course if the single-payer is the government it will most likely own the facilities themselves. There would be no manufacturer of pharmaceuticals, medical devices, or technology products that could afford to lose this single-payer entity as a customer. You can see from this the explanation for why these manufacturers sell the same items for a lot cheaper to other countries with public health systems.

3. Create a uniform Electronic Health Record platform, which would essentially provide an almost instantaneous cure for the fragmentation of hospital systems. The extra cost related to the lack of communication between doctors would be eliminated. This would have enormous money-saving and life-saving advantages.

4. Design and implement the standardization of medical decision-making. The entity would have the authority to design and oversee the implementation of the standardizing care scoring methods that will be described in the next chapter. As you have already seen, the subjectivity of the medical decision-making process is a key contributor to excessive health care costs as well as to poorer outcomes of treatment.

5. Implement a doctor compensation program to replace the fee-for-service system, with its inherent pitfalls both in terms of costs and treatment outcomes. Remember that the fee-for-service system rewards doctors for higher volumes of treatment, regardless of the effectiveness. Under this proposed compensation program, on the other hand, doctors would be salaried employees. Their salary and bonuses could be derived using the resource-based relative value scale (RBRVS) system created by the American Medical Association, which assigns a relative value to work done by doctors (the relative value assessment incorporates

factors like technical skill required, amount of time taken, and amount of effort required). Under this system, doctors work a certain number of relative value units, or RVUs. The better the treatment outcomes and patient satisfaction levels, the more patients will seek treatment by that doctor, resulting in more RVUs. Crucially, employers can reward better outcomes and satisfaction levels by increasing the doctor's earnings per RVU worked. If the single-payer is the government, employment of doctors under this system would be mandatory.

There are several other advantages, but these are the most obvious ones. There is no entity or group of entities that will be able to deliver these crucial remedies unless it is either the government or a single entity with government-like authority.

As you will see in Chapter 22, Obamacare may have slowed the rate of increase in the government component of health expenditure, but it resulted in a significant increase in the private component (the expenditures by individuals and employers through health insurance companies). Because health insurance companies are for-profit, they largely shifted the cost burden onto the insured, which means individuals pay higher premiums, co-payments (payments made by a person for a service, in addition to the insurance), co-insurance, and deductibles, in addition to paying for items no longer covered. A single-payer system is the only solution to tackle both government and private health care expenditures in one fell swoop. It is no wonder that other OECD countries with public health systems spend far less than us and provide their citizens with better health care results. And this reduced spending leads to benefits for all levels of American society: the government will have a reduced deficit, corporations will have more profits and ability to employ people, and individuals and families will have an increased standard of living (due to significant savings compared to what they spend on health care today).

Cutting Out the Middlemen
The single-payer system will dramatically reduce the need for, and the costs of, middlemen (health insurance companies and medical billing companies) because providers will be paid directly by that one single-payer entity. So, neither insurance nor medical billing companies are necessary in this system.

Many will argue that cutting out these two middlemen will increase unemployment. However, this is a superficial way to look at the situation. Indeed, there will inevitably be higher unemployment in the short-term because of the job cuts in these two sectors. This unemployment is the "short-term pain" which will be certainly be followed by "long-term gain," as capital and labor is freed up to be deployed to the productive part of the economy. One can easily argue that the money saved by citizens from high insurance premiums, co-payments, deductibles, and co-insurance will be freed up to spur economic activity as consumers spend it on goods and services. Remember that there will also be cost savings for corporations, which helps them to be more profitable and to expand and hire more employees. Additionally, there will be savings for the government, which can help decrease deficits. It is a virtuous cycle. These savings for individuals, corporations, and the government would easily more than offset the decrease in income of the laid-off employees of health insurance and medical billing companies. As discussed, the standard of living of any nation is based not on consumption but on increased production and productivity in the long run. Long-term gains are always worth the comparatively small short-term pains – in medicine, in economics, and in life!

Another Seemingly "Too Good To Be True" Scenario – An Example from a Public Health System
In the British public system of health care, there is another key benefit of having a sole payer. The British system can afford to have at least four generalist doctors of varying degrees of seniority take care of each patient admitted to every hospital (and five doctors at teaching hospitals). All of these physicians see the same

patient and make a collective decision, unlike in the U.S. where ONE generalist doctor (a "hospitalist") has the sole say in inpatient care, except in teaching hospitals.

As a doctor for almost four decades in both systems, I cannot convey to you how reassuring this system of collective decision-making is. A decision comes from four doctors of varying degrees of seniority (the house officer, senior house officer, registrar, and consultant), each with a different set of "dimensions" (recall, the "Four Dimensions" are knowledge, training, experience and judgment). And these four general doctors do not count the other specialists involved in caring for the patient within their specific specialties. It is impossible to put proper value on the pooling of the minds that happens here. Four doctors with different levels of seniority seeing the same patients is reassuring for both the patients and the doctors. With this system of checks and balances, a major mistake or omission is incredibly unlikely to happen. If one doctor made an error, it would be caught and corrected by another, and another, and yet another! And when a patient is in the hospital, usually considerably sicker than patients treated in outpatient settings, this safeguard means their lives, pure and simple.

Financing this Entity (if the entity is not the government)
This area is beyond my expertise as a doctor and I defer to the experts in health care administration for the details. However, I will mention some potential sources of financing this single-payer. One source of financing can be money allocated to Medicare and Medicaid, as well as other government programs. The contributions made by employers to fund their employees' health insurance as well as the premiums from individuals directly can also be used. The amount of money allocated should be determined by the enlisted population of a given unit, which will be discussed later under the suggested pilot program. As you can already sense, the financing aspect is complicated, and it is one reason to keep it simple and have the government as the single-payer.

Closing Thoughts on the Need For a Single-Payer System
There is no doubt that this suggestion is one that will take years to develop. I dearly hope that there may come a time when lawmakers will rise above politics and try to answer this simple question themselves: if we are spending more than any industrial nation on health care, why do we not have the health results to match? This is a fact, not an opinion. Is there something terribly wrong with the system? The answer to this question must be a logical "yes." Once a person, in this case a politician, sees the gravity of this problem, he or she must search for a solution, no matter the political costs or potential unpopularity. So, I hold out hope that our lawmakers will have the fortitude to make such a change, and that the American people will push them to take action to protect our health and lives.

CHAPTER EIGHTEEN
STANDARDIZE MEDICAL DECISION-MAKING

I advocate creating a more standardized model of medical decision-making that holds doctors and hospitals accountable by a numeric system. The numeric score comes as close as possible to uniform decision-making. The objective is to attach numeric values to diagnostic tests and procedures as well as medical and surgical treatment modalities. The values will be based on effectiveness, relative cost, and patient-specific factors. Essentially, this helps allocate finite resources more efficiently. This is perhaps the most difficult remedy both to present and to implement, but it will be crucial in ensuring cost effective treatment, will markedly decrease unnecessary surgery and procedures, and will make unnecessary expenses unlikely.

Difficult to Present
Unless you are a physician and an economist at the same time, or at least a physician with a good knowledge of economics, you may be likely to call these proposals health care "rationing," with the evil connotations that commonly go with the word. This is a prime example of how journalistic sensationalism and political demagoguery prey on people's lack of knowledge about a topic. Because of this, the solution can be difficult to present.

As we concluded in the chapter on economics, health care resources are finite. What we will attempt to do here is create a framework to allocate these finite resources: (1) to effective modalities of treatment; and (2) to go where most needed.

Sensationalists will not only call this "evil rationing" of

health care, but they will also cloud the conversation and paralyze a rational-thinking individual from finding a solution. You may find a headline like this: "Rationing is absolutely unacceptable! Only God can determine who lives and who dies!" A statement like that serves to stir emotions and manipulate the discussion to prevent you from using proper reasoning. Recall the example of the 95 year-old Australian woman with Alzheimer's who needed a hip replacement at the same time that her great grandson needed a kidney transplant to survive. If the family has a limited supply of money and can only treat one member, it must choose. Think about this as if it is your own family and you are the one to choose.

Remember, this example of a family with limited health care funds is a microcosm of the nation. Thankfully, by this part of the book, we are well equipped to see through any sensationalism and rationally analyze this potential remedy.

Difficult to Implement
Even if we create well-crafted numerical proposals to standardize medical decision-making, there will still be remaining subjectivity in gauging these numbers. It is impossible to eliminate all subjectivity, as medicine is not an exact science and medical decision-making is inherently subjective. Nevertheless, it is a much-needed attempt to bridge the enormous gaps in medical decision-making due to the variance in physicians' "Four Dimensions," as we have discussed. If there were a standard designed by experts, based on evidence and with numbers attached to it, there would be some uniformity and far less deviation from that standard. The standard created by this method would be credible and enforceable by one entity with authority. Those are two attributes that we do not have today, and they are sorely needed.

An Indisputable Need
Though medical decision-making is highly subjective both in choice of diagnostic tools and – more significantly – of treatment, there is no reason why some entity (that is authorized with the necessary power) cannot craft some much-needed standards

according to evidence-based medicine. As we know, doctors and patients do not fully take into account cost in their current decision-making, so there is a need for uniform decision-making guidelines about the most cost-effective diagnostic tools and treatment modalities. In other words, we absolutely need a "standard."

So, I will present some of my ideas on how to most effectively implement such standardization.

Crafting the Standards

Before you decide to consider standardized numeric scoring as a form of "evil rationing" of health care resources, I must remind you that:

1. As we saw in the Introduction, the U.S. is already spending an enormous percentage (about 17 percent) of our GDP on health care while Americans are less healthy than others around the world.

2. Health care resources are finite. One treatment takes away from all others. This is simply how resources are; if they were unlimited, as we all wish they were, there would be no need to have this discussion.

If you agree with these two statements, we can move forward in discussing the implementation of this much-needed standardization. A panel of leading medical, health care administration, and medical ethics experts can establish numeric scores that can be used by medical practitioners and can be enforced by the to-be-created single-payer entity. In this way, whether you are an American physician running a small practice in a rural area or operating in a massive research university hospital, you are abiding by the same rules and being held accountable.

Arriving at Numeric Scores

As mentioned, the three factors that need to be inputs into our analysis are: effectiveness, cost, and the particular case of the patient.

1. *The effectiveness of a diagnostic tool or treatment.* An example of a numeric scoring system for this would be giving a +100 score for the treatments that have been proven most effective from available evidence and giving a -100 score for the treatments proven to be least effective. This will allow a better understanding of what treatments have been proven effective and helpful to patients and what treatments have not. An effective diagnostic test for a broken bone, for example, is an X-ray. An effective test for a gall bladder stone is an ultrasound. In the case of treating bacterial pneumonia, the most effective treatments are appropriate antibiotics. For inguinal hernia, the most effective treatment is surgery. These numeric scores would allow a more-than-anecdotal analysis of effectiveness. The scores would be determined by an expert panel of doctors experienced in each area of medicine or surgery, and this panel would meet periodically to update the scores in light of advances in medicine and surgery, as well as to update the effectiveness of treatments accordingly.

2. *The cost.* The higher the cost of the diagnostic test or treatment, the worse the score should be, and vice versa. Again, we can use the -100 to +100 scale. Treating pneumonia by antibiotic – which would have already received the highest score on effectiveness – would have the highest score on this metric as well, while a heart-lung transplant would receive the most negative score in this category. These scores would be determined by an expert panel of health care administrators who would meet periodically to update the cost of diagnostic tools and treatment modalities.

3. *The patient.* Unlike the other two factors, this factor will be

determined by the physician on a case-by-case basis. The physician will depend on guidance from a panel of leading medical ethicists, including numeric scoring based on several patient-specific factors. These factors include the patient's age, associated diseases, and more. Remember the example I gave earlier of the great-grandmother who had Alzheimer's and multiple previous strokes. Because of these background factors, her surgery would score on the lower end because of its many possible negative repercussions. Her great grandson, who desperately needed the kidney transplant to live beyond early childhood, would score higher on the scale. This third factor – the set of patient-specific factors – can also be given a score of -100 to +100.

Putting the Factors Together and Making a Decision
These three factors must be considered together and weighed in light of one another. Treatments like a heart-lung transplant would probably score at the lowest level for having very little proven effectiveness and being very expensive. It is likely that patient-specific factors would only make this treatment even more dangerous and less desirable. By the same token, treating bacterial pneumonia with antibiotics would probably score the highest because it is cheap and very effective. A kidney transplant in a child born with polycystic kidney would have a reasonably good score because of the effectiveness of the surgery and the age of the patient, despite being expensive. On the other hand, the hip replacement for the elderly individual with Alzheimer's would score low because of the high costs and the patient-specific factors, despite the effectiveness of the surgery. I hope that these examples illustrate to you how the scoring system would work.

Again, demagogues will call this "evil rationing" to stir your emotions, but now you know it is not. It is a common sense approach to putting the finite resources of health care dollars where they are most effective and most needed.

The Benefits of Standardization
Use of this scoring system will make decisions as uniform as possible from one locality to another and from one provider to another regardless of doctors' opinions, which we have concluded are highly subjective and differ widely. This is not taking away the autonomy of the treating physician or surgeon; it is simply a tool to smooth out the sometimes dramatic divergences of opinion. It is another layer of protection for the patient – a structured second opinion based on evidence.

CHAPTER NINETEEN
IMPROVE TRAINING OF PRIMARY CARE PHYSICIANS TO BE THE ANCHORS OF HEALTH CARE

This is perhaps the least obvious to those who have tried to correct what is ailing the system and also the most promising in the long run. It will take several years to reap the benefits of implementing this suggestion.

Improved Training of PCPs
As we have discussed, primary care physicians play an absolutely crucial role in the health care system. I like to say that primary care is at the heart of the health care delivery system. It is the fulcrum around which all the players in the health care system revolve. All things start and end with the primary care physician.

As we discussed in detail in Chapter 6, the PCP has a critical and widely-encompassing role. So it is imperative that the training of primary care physicians be top-notch. In my opinion, this may be the single most important factor in making health care more efficient and of better quality.

A well-trained PCP, in terms of the three primary dimensions of the "making of a doctor" that we discussed in Chapter 3 (knowledge, training, and experience), is key. To obtain this, PCPs should be trained longer and in more areas of medicine. I advocate that medical schools implement a five-year residency in primary care. Almost all of that time should be spent in outpatient facilities, not in hospitals. This is because of the fact that the recent emergence of hospitalists as a specialty in medicine has made PCP training in a hospital setting largely unnecessary. Finally, it may be a good idea to give these future primary care physicians a course on the economics of health care so they better understand the implications of their decisions and actions on the larger system itself.

Ideally, this new, better-trained class of primary care physicians will order tests only when well-targeted. They will be able to manage more of the need of the patient without excessive consultation. They will possess a widened scope of education to know and do more without unnecessary referrals to specialists.

The Rise of "Physician Extenders"
The erroneous belief that physician extenders (nurse practitioners and physician assistants) can replace a well-trained PCP with less cost is a short-sighted and faulty assumption, as quite the opposite happens when they are utilized in the primary care setting.

Sixteen years ago, I wrote an editorial published in our local professional journal, *Northeast Florida Medicine* (then called *Jacksonville Medicine*), entitled "A Health Care Utopia!?: Making the Case for Creating a New Kind of Training for a New Breed of Physicians." In this editorial, I advocated – as I am in this book – training PCPs longer and in various aspects to know more and to do more. Since that time, sadly, the reverse has happened, as a good deal of physician extenders are left to make the decisions to test and refer to specialists. This substitution, in many ways, plays an important part in health care cost increases. The role of physician extenders is not at all to be a substitute for a competent PCP. These physician extenders, by comparison, are deficient in the first three dimensions discussed.

So, rather than investing in better training for more and higher caliber primary care physicians, we have gone down a route of surrounding existing PCPs with assistants who, though they are helpful in a specialist setting, can be costly in the primary care setting. They are simply no replacement for PCPs. In my opinion, physician extenders' roles should be limited to non-primary care areas in which there is less autonomy. As we have discussed, a sound set of "Four Dimensions" in a primary care provider is crucial in avoiding unnecessary costs related to excessive testing, excessive prescribing, and excessive specialist referrals.

A Well-Trained PCP is Indispensable
We have already seen an example of a poor decision at the primary care provider level that caused huge duress and enormous expenses for a patient when we discussed the case of Joanne in Chapter 4. If you remember, Joanne's provider was a physician extender who followed a spot on her chest X-ray for a longer time than was warranted, resulting in a chain of three different specialist visits (to a radiologist, a pulmonologist, and a thoracic surgeon) and two invasive procedures and surgeries that placed Joanne in an intensive care unit for days and could have easily taken her life. In the end, the spot on the X-ray was simply a scar. Hundreds of thousands of dollars were wasted, and a life could have been lost.

Clearly, for the sake of the efficiency of the system and the health of patients, we need to empower and equip PCPs to reliably and confidently handle their patients' needs. A well-trained PCP saves money and lives.

CHAPTER TWENTY
IMPLEMENT MEDICAL MALPRACTICE REFORM

Malpractice reform, in my view, is crucial to reducing defensive testing, which was mentioned before as one of the causes of excessive testing. There is an old adage in medicine: "When you hear hoof beats, think of horses, not zebras." While the source of the hoof beats can in fact be a zebra, and that should certainly be considered, it is the far less likely source. Many doctors are too preoccupied with avoiding malpractice suits; they perform several expensive tests, even when the clinical picture does not warrant these tests, just to make sure that all possible liability has been removed from them. They look – even search – for a zebra as opposed to looking for the more likely horse.

First of all, to avoid frivolous suits, there should be a requirement that, in order to move forward with a case of malpractice, one's case go through the scrutiny of medical professionals. If a case does go forward, it should be tried by a panel of judges rather than the jury system. Medical malpractice cases are always complex. At the heart of it, there is a good deal of mathematics and odds that the average juror is not equipped to understand. The judges should be able to understand the inexact nature of medicine that we have discussed. Additionally, the judges should be able to grasp the "reasonable" risk in the face of treating a condition that – in many cases – has a certain bad outcome that is coming if there is no treatment.

It is very reasonable to expect the judges who are determining malpractice cases to have a strong understanding of the practice of medicine. After all, these judges are determining whether or not a doctor appropriately or inappropriately acted in the face of a complex, stressful, and uncertain situation. The trial attorneys who often take advantage of the complexity of the situation and the statistics surrounding it to improperly sway a jury will not sway these highly competent judges.

The good news is that the malpractice environment has improved recently, and reform has been accomplished before to make a positive change (though not in the ways I describe). As Stanford University professor Dr. Michelle Mello said after conducting an analysis of paid malpractice claims over time, "after years of turbulence, the medical liability environment has calmed."[1] In terms of models for reform, we can consider Texas. There, reforms were made that resulted in improvements in the system of hearing malpractice cases. In 2003, the Texas legislature capped damages in the state's medical malpractice lawsuits. A little over 10 years later, the Department of Insurance data shows that medical malpractice claims resolved in a year fell by nearly two-thirds between 2003 and 2011. The average payout also declined by 22 percent. This "tort reform" has allowed doctors to be a bit less concerned about being sued (from a place where they were far too concerned, in my opinion) and to have lower malpractice insurance premiums, which cuts down on health care costs.[2]

CHAPTER TWENTY-ONE
A PILOT PROGRAM: IMPLEMENT SELF-CONTAINED COMMUNITY HEALTH CENTERS

Even if the country chooses public health, it will be difficult to execute the shift to a public health system in less than 7 to 10 years. The pilot program suggested here can be used as a model throughout the country after trying it for a few years on a smaller scale. This pilot program can only be implemented in an urban setting with at least two (the more, the better) competing hospital systems.

How SCCHCs are Formed
To improve communication and competition among physicians and hospitals, I advocate creating what I call Self-Contained Community Health Centers, or SCCHCs. Within a reasonable distance from a hospital, the other components of the SCCHC will be found. These components will include PCPs and specialists, as well as ancillary health care facilities. All of these components will be integrated with the hospital around which the SCCHC is formed. Every member within this SCCHC will have access to everything being done to a patient (all tests and treatments) within its boundaries. Patients will choose which SCCHC to initially enroll in based on their preference in terms of PCP, hospital, existing provider, and other factors. The money allocated to each SCCHC will be based on how many patients are enrolled in it. That money will be derived from all sources related to the enrolled patients' insurances, whether private or government funded.

The success of each SCCHC unit will depend on an evaluation of two factors:

1. The number of patients who choose to enroll in the SCCHC. As mentioned, this will be based on the patients' preference for any of the SCCHC's components (the hospital itself or the PCPs and/or specialists assigned to this unit). The number of enrolled patients will determine the amount of money the SCCHC will receive. If the patient is currently enrolled in Medicaid or Medicare, these two entities will pay each SCCHC a certain amount of money per patient per month, which will be applied to all of its elements (the hospital, ancillary health services, and doctors within the unit). Patients who are currently insured by commercial insurance, whether directly or through their employer, can pay premiums directly to the SCCHC, which will function as the provider of services as well as the insurer. Of course, for a given SCCHC, the better the outcomes of its treatments and the more patients that are satisfied with it, the more people will enroll and thus the more funds it will receive. It is worth noting that although this project is implemented at the local and state level, it is federally created and thus federal insurance funding to these units is assured.

2. How efficient that SCCHC is in regards to spending its allocated funds for the services it provides.

Finally, doctors assigned to each unit would be salaried employees with bonuses given according to both patient satisfaction and treatment outcomes.

Ensuring Accountability and Fostering Competition
The SCCHC as a unit – a kind of health care hub – will be helpful in assessing the quality of care by health care players as one unit (hospitals, PCPs, specialists, and ancillary health care facilities). The

quality of care provided by these units will be graded, and this information will be visible to all. The better quality of care and the better the outcome statistics (including patient satisfaction), the more patients that the SCCHC will attract, the more money that will flow into it, and the more successful the SCCHC will be. This creates accountability among practitioners and also allows for patient-focused incentivisation.

The transparency of this structure will foster competition among SCCHCs because patients will be able to seamlessly move from one SCCHC to another if they are unsatisfied with their PCPs, specialists, or hospital. This way, there will be some mobility from one SCCHC to another, but the fragmentation of health information and duplicate services will be minimal. The entity that shrinks due to unfavorable preferences and patients moving will be forced to keep examining and reexamining the reasons behind their problems and to correct them in order to better cater to patients. If they do not, the whole management of the system may be handed over to another, more successful SCCHC.

A single-payer system is necessary for this process to work. Indeed, this actually conveys how a single-payer system will create a greater element of competition, as in the free market place. For those who fear a government-run system, this model can serve as an alternative with inherent competition built in, enough to reward excellence for those who meet the goals of delivering high quality and affordable health care. Also, this suggestion will allay the fears of those politicians on the conservative end of the political spectrum. So, in reality, what is called "socialism" by so many would actually improve free market competition. I told you not to succumb to journalistic sensationalism and political demagoguery!

Improving Communication
Crucially, the SCCHCs should each have the same digital platform of Electronic Health Records. The systems must be unified so that access to all information about patients can be available to any provider who needs that information within minutes. Just imagine the redundancies and inefficiencies that this would eliminate! As

mentioned in Chapter 10, the CPRS system adopted by the Veterans Health Administration is a great example of unified EHR. Any practitioner in any department can easily pull up a patient's name and find all of his or her records from all of his or her various visits to the hospital, including all scans and bloodwork. Not only does this cut down on duplicate testing, but it also allows each practitioner to have a greater understanding of the patient's condition as a whole. Unifying EHR would significantly increase both efficiency and quality of care.

Implementing SCCHCs
The creation of SCCHCs would significantly decrease the unnecessary repeated tests and streamline management of patients' health. This suggestion would be a major treatment for the fragmented and wasteful elements of the health care system that we have discussed.

In my opinion, this idea is worth trying as a pilot program in a city first. It cures many of the underlying inefficiencies and high costs of the system, but, as I mentioned, it can only be implemented under a single-payer system (which does not exist anywhere in the U.S. currently). Ultimately, this SCCHC model can be a final system of delivering health care if the pilot program proves to be successful, or perhaps it can serve as a transitional model en route to a more centralized one.

SECTION VI.
A CALL TO ACTION

There we have it: a look at some of the most pressing problems with the American health care system and some of the solutions that myself and others find to be the most promising. With an understanding of all this, we are each uniquely equipped to help cure this ailing system to ensure people have the joy and peace of quality and affordable health care. We are each capable of moving forward with the prescription and beginning the healing.

We are at a special time in history, indeed. It is one in which health care discussion dominates the conversation through the ongoing implementation and second-guessing of Obamacare. It is one in which a new generation of young people is entering the workforce in place of the retiring Baby Boomers. And it is one in which the nation is becoming more frustrated with its mounting debt and more cognizant that something must change to ensure a strong and sustainable economic future.

As we launch forward to make a change, we must dig into the past that has led us to this point and then consider the urgency of this particular moment in time.

CHAPTER TWENTY-TWO
FROM TEDDY ROOSEVELT TO BARACK OBAMA AND BEYOND: THE QUEST FOR UNIVERSAL, AFFORDABLE HEALTH CARE CONTINUES

Of course, our generation is not the first to grapple with debates about what to do with American health care. As we discussed from the beginning, we all have at least one thing in common: health care is critically important to our lives. This has been true and will remain true. For the past 100 years, the American discussion on health care has evolved and developed. Before we move forward to a hopefully brighter future of solutions and cost-effectiveness, it is important to briefly understand where we came from.

This history of mostly failed calls for reform to create universal health coverage for all people – from the presidencies of Teddy Roosevelt to Barack Obama – shows how U.S. health policy has come to be where it is today. These events have left us with, as Jonathan Oberlander puts it, "a patchwork of public and private coverage."[1]

As we will see in tracing the history of reform (largely adapted from the Kaiser Family Foundation's "History of Health Reform in the U.S." timeline and from Oberlander's article in *The New England Journal of Medicine*), reform ideas that aligned with one party actually ended up becoming entrenched positions of the other, and vice versa. Leaders of both parties have advocated universal health coverage at different moments in history. Groups that once supported certain ideas became detractors later on. This yet again underscores that we cannot look at this through a partisan lens if we truly wish to find solutions. The health of the American people cannot be a political prop.

Theodore Roosevelt's Progressive Party
Just a bit over 100 years ago, President Theodore Roosevelt and his party proposed social insurance as a part of its platform, and that included health insurance. In 1915, a bill for compulsory health insurance was drafted by the American Association for Labor Legislation (AALL), and a few states were interested. The American Medical Association initially supported the plan, though it would later reverse its support. The idea was to follow in the footsteps of European nations, like the U.K. and Germany, in ensuring medical care for all workers.[2]

Ultimately, World War I, which began in 1914, helped create a pause in that discussion. Serious opposition from primarily businesses and insurance companies played a role in the failure of the reform efforts, as did the political demagoguery that we have discussed as a factor in today's debate. Anti-German sentiment was pervasive during this time, and government-commissioned articles vilified "German socialist insurance."[3] Opponents of reform called the proposals for universal care "un-American," among other labels intended to sway the public against the idea.[4] Indeed, the same obstacles that exist today existed 100 years ago. Not much has changed in that regard.

The Great Depression, FDR, and the New Deal
The difficult economic times of the Great Depression led to President Franklin Delano Roosevelt's focus on expanding social policies to create safety nets for Americans. This package of social policy programs was called the "New Deal," as it was meant to bring about a new deal or agreement with the American people. In the end, FDR's Committee on Economic Security decided not to include national health reform in the landmark Social Security Act because of fear that it would put the bill's passage at risk.[5]

By the 1940s, the proposals moved from calling for health insurance for all workers to calling for health insurance for all people: universal health coverage. In FDR's second term, there was a renewed push for national health insurance after the Social Security Act passed. In his 1944 State of the Union address, FDR outlined the "economic bill of rights," in which he included the right to adequate medical care and the opportunity to achieve and enjoy good health. Senator Robert Wagner introduced the National Health Act of 1939, which would give states greater provisions, through federal grants, to provide public health. But, with a Congress that was not supportive of further government expansions, universal coverage would not yet come.[6] Employer-sponsored private insurance, instead, began covering Americans more and more in the 1940s and 1950s as unions pressed their employers to provide health support. The federal government, in turn, subsidized employer-sponsored coverage by allowing tax exclusions. Employer-sponsored health insurance remained an incomplete solution to providing care for all people.[7]

President Truman and the Fair Deal
Shortly after the end of World War II in 1945, President Harry S. Truman was the next president to push for a national health program, and this time it seemed entirely inevitable. His election seemed to be a mandate for national health insurance. Truman proposed a single egalitarian system that encompassed all of society. The American Medical Association strongly opposed this, fearing it would make slaves of doctors. Republicans, who took control of Congress in 1946, referred to this as "socialized medicine," linking it with communist thought.[8] Southern Democrats also opposed the idea, fearing that a federal role in health care may require desegregation.[9] Again, we see the effort towards a national health program was thwarted by many of the same factors that contributed to the failure of the Progressives decades prior.

Lyndon Johnson and the Great Society
As employer-based health coverage grew in the late 1950s and early 1960s, private plans began setting premiums based on their newfound understanding of health costs. This meant that

affordable health coverage was difficult to find for the disabled and the retired. In response to this, President John F. Kennedy addressed the nation on the idea of Medicare, a social insurance program for the elderly, in Madison Square Garden in 1962. President Lyndon Johnson, who assumed the presidency in 1963 after Kennedy's assassination, then advocated Medicare in a special message to Congress in 1964. In 1965, President Johnson presided over the creation of Medicare as well as Medicaid, a social insurance program for the low-income, as part of the Social Security Act. Former President Truman was there by his side as he signed the bill in July of 1965.[10]

These landmark federal health insurance programs are certainly two of the most significant reforms in health care in the 20th century. They came about due to Johnson's political abilities, a favorable Congressional environment, the support of the hospitals and insurance companies, and – crucially – the support of the public.[11] It would prove to be difficult to find such aligning stars again.

This enactment of Medicare and Medicaid is an example of the new strategy of reformers. Seeing that attempts at gaining comprehensive health insurance were not working, reformers from the mid-20th century onward have focused on expanding coverage for particular demographic groups one at a time, including the elderly, the poor, pregnant women, children, persons with disabilities, and persons with specific illnesses.[12]

An Era of Disagreement, Kicking the Can Down the Road, and Growing Concern About Costs
Still, this piecemeal approach left significant gaps in coverage. After the breakthrough of the agreement that led to Medicare and Medicaid, the United States saw a period of continued disagreement when it came to health care. It is one that has lasted, regrettably, all the way through the present.

In 1969, Democratic Senator Ted Kennedy first called for a comprehensive national health insurance program, and he continued his pursuit of it for his entire career. He proposed the

Health Security Act, calling for a universal single-payer plan financed through payroll taxes. Republican President Richard Nixon proposed his own plan. His Comprehensive Health Insurance Plan "called for universal coverage, voluntary employer participation, and a separate program for the working poor and the unemployed, replacing Medicaid."[13] Though they came close to reaching an agreement, Kennedy ultimately did not back Nixon's plan. With the Watergate hearings and President Nixon's resignation, comprehensive health insurance took a backseat.[14] However, Nixon was able to expand Medicare eligibility to cover those under the age of 65 with long-term disabilities and those with end-stage renal disease in 1972.

Proposals to improve the quality of health care for all Americans were overshadowed by a dark spot in American history. The conversation about health care was drowned out by the scandal engulfing the White House under Nixon. This would happen yet again, as Republican President Gerald Ford supported national health reform, with Representative Wilbur Mills drafting a compromise bill. This bill stalled, largely as Mills faced a personal scandal that forced him to leave Congress.[15]

Next, President Jimmy Carter – a Democrat from Georgia – moved to tackle the growing health care costs and need for improved quality and greater coverage. He focused largely on the cost side, however, and prioritized cost containment over expanding coverage of care. Senator Kennedy came back with another national health insurance plan, but everything stalled yet again in the midst of an economic recession.[16]

President Bill Clinton's energy showed promise for something to get done to improve our ailing health care system. He proposed a "managed competition" approach, which called for universal coverage, an individual mandate to have insurance, competition among insurers, and government regulation to reduce costs. Powerful interests – namely the Health Insurance Association of America and the National Federation of Independent Businesses – fought the bill, Congress was divided, and the progress halted. But all was not lost; in 1997, the Children's

Health Insurance Program was created, building on the Medicaid program by providing health care coverage for children of low-income families that do not qualify for Medicaid.[17]

Meanwhile, outside of the halls of government, Americans suffered. Many Americans without employer-based coverage could not afford to purchase comprehensive health insurance. Health care costs grew and, as a result of the lack of affordability, the uninsured population in the U.S. grew from 31 million (12.9 percent of the population) to 50 million (16.3 percent of the population) just between 1987 and 2010.[18]

This era did see perhaps the beginning of the growing concern about health care costs in America. Nixon implemented price controls on the health care industry and promoted health maintenance organizations (HMOs); Congress under President Ford aimed to rationalize resource use through certificate-of-need requirements; Carter had a failed plan to contain hospital costs; Congress under the first President Bush enacted a Medicare fee schedule.[19] Yet costs continued to grow dramatically as these controls usually only applied to the federal system, not to the health care system as a whole. As we will see in the next chapter, these costs are one reason why we must act now to find solutions for our system of health.

President Obama and Obamacare
The quest for universal coverage and some sort of way to stop the cost bleeding eventually ended up in the hands of President Barack Obama. After a prolonged and bitter battle, the Patient Protection and Affordable Care Act (ACA) – more commonly known as Obamacare – was signed in 2010.

This historic legislation made, and is in the process of making, a few significant changes in terms of expanding health insurance availability and access to care. For one, it requires that all individuals obtain health insurance coverage (the individual mandate). Those who do not obtain "minimum essential coverage" throughout the year and are not exempt must pay a fee (an Individual Shared Responsibility Payment). There is also an employer mandate that requires large employers to provide coverage for full-time employees, or pay a penalty (Employer Shared Responsibility Payment). The ACA created state-based health insurance exchanges, or marketplaces, that allow Americans without health insurance to shop for coverage and see if they are eligible for subsidies. Additionally, the ACA prevents insurers from discriminating against those with pre-existing conditions or putting lifetime limits on coverage. The ACA also allows individuals to stay on their parents' health insurance until age 26, regardless of whether they are dependents for tax purposes.[20]

The Century-Long Wait Continues: The Obamacare Illusion
While Obamacare was meant to ensure accessibility of health coverage, it still falls short of universal coverage and does not include any of the recommendations in this book to improve quality and decrease costs of care. As Oberlander points out, even if the Affordable Care Act reaches its target of covering 30 million uninsured people by the time it is fully implemented, this will still mean that 30 million people will remain uninsured 10 years from now.[21]

Journalist Jennifer Rubin of *The Washington Post* summed up Obamacare in this manner: "Practically nothing about Obamacare is turning out to be what President Obama said it would be."[22] Even though this extreme characterization may be politically-charged, the conclusion is substantially true. While Obamacare has proven to reduce the number of uninsured Americans,[23] it seems to have come at the expense of the insured. Crucially, individual premiums have increased for many (even judging from my own conversations with patients) and may increase by up to a third, with spillover to employer-sponsored insurance premiums.[24] So many families with modest incomes cannot afford family coverage offered by their employers and are essentially priced out of the market, even though they afforded it before. In other words, poor and low-income patients who could not have health insurance before Obamacare are able to get it because of government subsidies; however, they are displacing the ones who were able to pay for insurance previously, but are now unable to afford it or can only afford the premiums of insurance plans with very high deductibles and/or high co-insurance. This is a quickly expanding group that I call "the class of underinsured" under Obamacare. So much for universal coverage.

There are many experts who have examined Obamacare and concluded that it is not the solution. For example, Dr. John Geyman, Professor Emeritus in Family Medicine at the University of Washington School of Medicine and prolific writer on health care issues, wrote a book published in January 2015 entitled *How Obamacare is Unsustainable: Why We Need a Single-Payer Solution for All Americans*. In it, Dr. Geyman discusses the flaws of the Affordable Care Act and how the legislation thus far has failed to meet its primary goals. With Obamacare, we are back to the "band-aid approaches" described in the Introduction; we are left once again waiting for a sustainable solution to our country's health care crisis.

The financial burden of health care costs was shifted to have more weight on the insured through higher premiums, higher co-payments, higher co-insurance, payments for items no longer covered, and higher deductibles. Thus, health care costs as a percentage of Americans' income has gone up. Needless to say, this will decrease economic growth with less disposable income left to be spent on other goods and services. Sticking to the theme of economic growth, the employer mandate disincentivizes the growth of full-time employment. Employers often try to avoid health coverage for full-time workers, so they hire part-time workers instead.

This is among many other pitfalls. Obamacare may have slowed the rate of increase in the government component of health care cost, but it increased the cost significantly to the presumably more "insured" citizens. In his analysis in *TIME Magazine*, Steven Brill concluded: "Put simply, with Obamacare we've changed the rules related to who pays for what, but we haven't done much to change the prices we pay."[25] As a patient, you are the first to notice that shift to bear more of the health care costs; you do not have to wait for a news item, a research article, or a statistical claim to tell you that. You judge this from your own experience; you are the arbiter. From this you can see that the "affordable and universal" coverage under Obamacare is largely nothing but an illusion.

Again, it comes back to economics: slowing the rate of increase in health care expenditures by the government is certainly helpful for the issue of the government debt and liability. But if you decrease the government component of cost and shift it to private citizens, it will slow overall economic activity because – again – less money is left as disposable income for citizens. This, in turn, decreases spending on goods and services. If you add decreased citizen spending because of the burden of health care costs to the decreased full-time employment opportunities because of the employer mandate (especially for young individuals, who also are faced with the burden of student loans and increases in apartment rental rates, among other challenges), you can guarantee slow economic growth if not outright lingering recession. When economic growth slows down, tax receipts by the government decrease and spending on welfare programs increases, making the government deficit and debt grow larger. It is a vicious cycle, and nothing will correct this other than what is prescribed in Chapter 17 in the treatment section of this book. An effective single-payer system treats both problems with one fell swoop and, as hard to believe as it is, it will also improve metrics of health care quality!

Business as Usual is Not an Option
While there has been piecemeal progress over the past 100 years, health care reform has very clearly fallen short and failed the American people. This becomes crystal clear when we again look at the difference in how much we pay and what we get compared to other developed nations. We have the most expensive system by far on the planet, poor results in nearly all metrics, a remaining roughly 17 percent of the non-elderly population uninsured as of 2013,[26] and a population of insured people who still struggle mightily with the costs associated with premiums and medical bills. For all the debates over the past century, there is no debate about one thing today: Americans all over the country – again, even the

ones who are insured – are unfairly put in positions that make them one illness away from disaster. It is inhumane and unjust, and it should be intolerable to all of us.

CHAPTER TWENTY-THREE
NO TIME TO WAIT

Any American who suffers and cannot afford his or her health care is one too many. We must act on health care improvements right now with a keen sense of urgency, not just to ensure there are fewer struggling Americans, but also because the economy and well-being of our nation itself desperately depends on action.

Why is there such urgency on the national scale? Let us take a look.

Unsustainable Trend of Health Care Spending
Health care spending in the U.S. has more than doubled as a share of GDP over the last 30 years. And it is projected to double again by 2035.[1] If the trend of the last two to three decades continues, we will be in enormous, enormous trouble (truthfully, we are already in significant trouble). In fact, the U.S. Department of Health and Human Services projects that health care spending in the U.S. will reach $4.3 trillion by 2017, and the Congressional Budget Office projects that total spending on health care will increase to 25 percent of GDP in 2025 if no changes in federal law occur.[2]

These are, of course, only projections and extrapolations, with various assumptions being made. But all trends support the conclusion that, if the inaction and inability to compromise that have plagued the last 50 plus years of health care reform continue into the future, we will have dug a massive hole and it will be very painful to climb out.

If they are not checked by new ideas, policies, and

initiatives, these rapidly rising costs will lead to far greater U.S. government spending on health care. Figure 23.1 on the following page shows projected federal spending on health care as a percentage of GDP.[3] Note that most of the increase in projected federal spending is the massive light grey section that represents excessive cost growth.

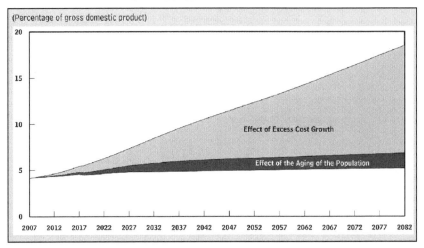

Figure 23.1
Sources of Growth in Projected Federal Spending on Medicare and Medicaid

Source: Congressional Budget Office

What is so striking, of course, is that this is only one side of the paradox we have discussed throughout this book: the paradox of paying more for health care and getting less. Sadly, with all of these expenditures and the unfettered growth, Americans are still receiving worse health care than most other developed nations that spend so much less. These costs are uncontrollable and unsustainable regardless, but the fact that they still lead to a lack of quality care means that they add – very literally – insult to injury.

Unsustainable Debt
Why does this increase in government spending matter so much? Firstly, of course, this is our money that is being taxed. On a macro level, this greater cost burden for our government only entrenches

our nation further into debt. Our government's total debt is nearing $19 trillion and continues to grow. That comes to nearly $60,000 for every citizen in the U.S. As we discussed in Chapter 15, many economists, like Laurence Kotlikoff, estimate that the actual debt total – if you include all future unfunded liabilities of the government – is an almost incomprehensible $210 trillion, or about $656,000 for every citizen. In fact, Kotlikoff said in 2010, "The U.S. is bankrupt and we don't even know it." He based this opinion on an annual International Monetary Fund (IMF) report that examined the United States' fiscal state.[4] Whether directly through hiked taxes or more subtly through growing inflation (and thus decreasing purchasing power, or decreasing the value of our money), we as American citizens will be on the hook for fixing this problem that continues to grow unchecked.

Foregone Investments
As a note, this also means less ability for the government to invest in other crucial projects. When the government has invested in the future during the past few decades, we have seen it aid tremendous developments as significant as GPS technology, the Human Genome Project, and – of course – the Internet. Today, however, it is difficult to find room for government investments in the next generation of developments when health care costs alone make up over one-fifth of the budget and the cost of servicing our debt increases.

1,000+ Economists and Young People Are Ringing the Alarm Bells
They say that no two economists agree on anything, but Kotlikoff and over 1,200 economists – including 17 Nobel Laureates – from both major political parties agree on one thing for sure: America has serious long-term financial problems that need to be addressed right now. These economists are the supporters of the bipartisan Intergenerational Financial Obligations Reform Act, or the INFORM Act. In *The New York Times*, an open letter from this group to the President and Congress in 2013 read:

"Unless we begin to systematically measure and address our long-term fiscal imbalances, no government programs, be they maintaining our nation's military or paying Social Security benefits, will be secure."[5]

Read that one more time, and remember that – once again – over 1,000 prominent economists of all backgrounds and schools of thought agree on this, including 17 Nobel Laureates in economics. Oftentimes in politics and policy discussions, it is hard to figure out whether or not an argument is valid or has enough expert support. This is NOT one of those times. Though we know that economics is an inexact science of differing opinions, this is an overwhelming and convincing level of agreement.

The INFORM Act, if passed, would disclose the true size and intergenerational consequences of the country's fiscal imbalance by incorporating fiscal gap and generational accounting analysis in the annual budget process. It is endorsed by over 15,000 Millennials – members of today's young adult generation who will deal with the brunt of the problem that is continuing to spiral out of control.[6]

However, it is not just young people who will suffer; everyone is at risk. As the economists point out, not even Social Security benefits – which so many Baby Boomers are relying on for a livable retirement – are secure if our nation's finances continue to stay on the existing path.

You do not have to be a Nobel Prize-winning economist, or an economist at all, to know that our nation needs to make moves right now to decrease its debt sharply, for the sake of the nation as a whole and for the sake of each citizen.

CHAPTER TWENTY-FOUR
FULFILLING A CENTURY-LONG DREAM: RISING ABOVE POLITICS TO ACHIEVE UNIVERSAL, AFFORDABLE HEALTH CARE

It has been a long and winding road of health care reform and developments. Because of the constant discussion about Obamacare and consequently health care in general, we now have a momentous opportunity to act.

Though I imagine you have been trying to guess and may feel confident one way or the other, I do not align with either political party. I am a pragmatist. In this era of partisanship, we need pragmatism more than ever and in this topic just as much as in any other, if not more so. We must embrace workable ideas originating from either party. After all, as we have seen, political parties and various interest groups are changing their perspectives on these ideas over time anyways.

No, partisan politics will not solve this health care and financial crisis. It will take a willingness of our leaders to engage in genuine, often difficult conversations about what must change. It will take a resolve to look past special interest groups and solely focus on what is best for the physical, emotional, and financial well-being of common Americans.

Perhaps you are reading this and are having many doubts about the likelihood that this will happen. Confidence in government is at historic lows, so you would not be alone in having these doubts. This is precisely why each of us needs to stand up and be heard. We need to be able to look past the ideological cloud and see the problems and the necessary solutions clearly.

Ultimately, we as a nation must be knowledgeable about the subject, and we must be aware of what is happening to our health and to our nation. This book hopefully provided you with a great launchpad. You may not agree with all of the things written here, but you are certainly equipped with a strong understanding of the dynamics of the problems facing our health care system and our country. Additionally, you have read stories and statistics about what is going on with the health care of Americans all across the nation, and you have processed several proposed ideas for how to make a change. You also have your own experience as a patient, which is crucial. You are ready and able to drive change.

So speak up, both in everyday conversations and in pushing your governmental representatives. Stand up for the health of our kids, our parents, our brothers, and our sisters. The United States stands as an incredible experiment in democracy that has continued to bend towards greater justice and social safety for people in need. Thankfully, as we have discussed, so many of the solutions to the dramatically rising health care costs will also increase the quality and accessibility of health care to heal our citizens. What is needed now is for our country to muster up the courage to make those changes for the greater good. Today, we must take the long overdue steps to creating justice, and cost-effectiveness, in the world of health care. Crazy enough, the steps to do both of those are right in front of us.

The diagnosis has been made. Let us now rise above politics and treat this cancer inside us.

Let us do it for ourselves, our families, our future generations, and our country.

Let us begin today.

DYING OF HEALTH CARE

ENDNOTES

Chapter One

1　Total expenditure on health per capita. *Organisation for Economic Co-operation and Development, 2014.* <http://www.oecd-ilibrary.org/social-issues-migration-health/total-expenditure-on-health-per-capita_20758480-table2>

2　Ibid.

3　National Health Expenditures 2013 Highlights. *Centers for Medicare & Medicaid Services,* 2013. <http://www.cms.gov/Research-Statistics-Data-and-Systems/Statistics-Trends-and-Reports/NationalHealthExpendData/downloads/highlights.pdf>

4　Fox, Maggie. Healthcare system wastes up to $800 billion a year. *Reuters,* 2009. <http://www.reuters.com/article/2009/10/26/us-usa-healthcare-waste-idUSTRE59P0L320091026>

5　OECD Health Statistics 2014: How Does the United States Compare? *Organisation for Economic Co-operation and Development,* 2014. <http://www.oecd.org/unitedstates/Briefing-Note-UNITED-STATES-2014.pdf>

6　Ibid.

7　Davis, K, Stremikis, K, Squires, D, Schoen, C. Mirror, Mirror on the Wall, 2014 Update: How the U.S. Health Care System Compares Internationally. *The Commonwealth Fund,* 2014. <http://www.commonwealthfund.org/~/media/files/publications/fund-report/2014/jun/1755_davis_mirror_mirror_2014.pdf>

8　Health Systems: Improving Performance. *The World Health Organization – World Health Report,* 2000. <http://www.who.int/whr/2000/en/whr00_en.pdf?ua=1>

9　Ibid #5.

10   Hospital beds. *Organisation for Economic Co-operation and Development*, 2014. <http://www.oecd-ilibrary.org/social-issues-migration-health/hospital-beds_20758480-table5>

11   Ibid #5.

12   Ibid #5.

13   World Health Statistics 2014. *World Health Organization*, 2014. <http://apps.who.int/iris/bitstream/10665/112738/1/9789240692671_eng.pdf?ua=1>

14   The World Factbook. *Central Intelligence Agency*, 2014. <https://www.cia.gov/library/publications/the-world-factbook/rankorder/2102rank.html>

15   Competitiveness Rankings. *World Economic Forum*, 2014. <http://reports.weforum.org/global-competitiveness-report-2014-2015/rankings>

16   Ibid #14.

17   MacDorman, M, Matthews, T, Mohangoo, A, Zeitlin, J. International Comparisons of Infant Mortality and Related Factors: United States and Europe, 2010. *National Vital Statistics Report.* 63 (5), 2014. <http://www.cdc.gov/nchs/data/nvsr/nvsr63/nvsr63_05.pdf>

18   Ibid #15.

19   U.S. Burden of Disease Collaborators. The State of US Health, 1999-2010: Burden of Diseases, Injuries, and Risk Factors. *The Journal of the American Medical Association.* 310 (6): 591-606, 2013. <http://jama.jamanetwork.com/article.aspx?articleid=1710486>

20   Compare Your Country – Health Profile. *Organisation for Economic Co-operation and Development*, 2013. <http://www.compareyourcountry.org/health?cr=oecd&cr1=oecd&lg=en&page=0>

21   OECD Health Statistics 2013. *Organisation for Economic Co-operation and Development*, 2013. <http://www.oecd-ilibrary.org/social-issues-migration-health/health-at-a-glance-2013_health_glance-2013-en>

Chapter Two

1   LaMontagne, C. NerdWallet Health Finds Medical Bankruptcy Accounts for Majority of Personal Bankruptcies. *NerdWallet*, 2014. <http://www.nerdwallet.com/blog/health/2014/03/26/medical-bankruptcy>

2   Himmelstein, D, Thorne, D, Warren, E, Woolhandler, S. Medical Bankruptcy in the United States, 2007: Results of a National Study. *The American Journal of Medicine*. 122 (8): 741-746, 2009. <http://www.pnhp.org/new_bankruptcy_study/Bankruptcy-2009.pdf>

3   Pollitz, K, Cox, C, Lucia, K, Keith, K. Medical Debt Among People with Health Insurance. *The Henry J. Kaiser Family Foundation*, 2014. <http://kaiserfamilyfoundation.files.wordpress.com/2014/01/8537-medical-debt-among-people-with-health-insurance.pdf>

4   Meessen, B, Zhenzhong, Z, Van Damme, W, Devadasan, N, Criel, B, Bloom, G. Iatrogenic Poverty. *Tropical Medicine & International Health*. 8 (7); 581-584, 2003. <http://onlinelibrary.wiley.com/doi/10.1046/j.1365-3156.2003.01081.x/full>

5   Ibid #2.

6   Ibid #3, pg 6.

7   Ibid #3, pg 4.

8   The Market for Long-Term Care Insurance. *The National Bureau of Economic Research*. <http://www.nber.org/bah/winter05/w10989.html>

Chapter Three

1   Wysowski, D, Pitts, M, Beitz, J. Depression and Suicide in Patients Treated with Isotretinoin. *The New England Journal of Medicine*. 344 (6), 2001. <http://www.nejm.org/doi/full/10.1056/NEJM200102083440616>

Chapter Four

1 Mello, M, Chandra, A, Gawande, A, Studdert, D. National Costs of the Medical Liability System. *National Institute of Health.* 29 (9), 2010. <http://www.ncbi.nlm.nih.gov/pmc/articles/PMC3048809/>

2 Berenson, R, Rich, E. US Approaches to Physician Payment: The Deconstruction of Primary Care. *Journal of General Internal Medicine.* 25 (6), 2010 <http://www.ncbi.nlm.nih.gov/pmc/articles/PMC2869428/#CR12>

3 Canavan, C, West, J, Card, T. The Epidemiology of Irritable Bowel Syndrome. *Clinical Epidemiology.* 6: 71-80, 2014. <http://www. ncbi.nlm.nih.gov/pmc/articles/PMC3921083>

4 Arbab-Zadeh, A. Stress Testing and Non-invasive Coronary Angiography in Patients with Suspected Coronary Artery Disease: Time for a New Paradigm. *Heart International.* 7 (1): e2, 2012. <http://www.ncbi.nlm.nih.gov/pmc/articles/PMC3366298>

Chapter Five

1 Aitken, M, Kleinrock, M, Lyle, J, Caskey, L. Medicine Use and Shifting Costs of Healthcare: A Review of the Use of Medicines in the United States in 2013. *IMS Institute for Healthcare Informatics,* 2014. <http://www.imshealth.com/deployedfiles/imshealth/Global/Content/Corporate/IMS%20Health%20Institute/Reports/Secure/ IIHI_US_Use_of_Meds_for_2013.pdf>

2 Health, United States, 2013 with Special Feature on Prescription Drugs. *Center for Disease Control and Prevention,* 2014. Pg 21. <http://www.cdc.gov/nchs/data/hus/hus13.pdf>

3 Prescription Drug Trends. *The Henry J. Kaiser Family Foundation,* 2010. Pg 3. <http://kaiserfamilyfoundation.files.wordpress.com/2013/01/3057-08.pdf>

4   Gu, Q, Dillon, C, Burt, V. Prescription Drug Use Continues to Increase: U.S. Prescription Drug Data for 2007-2008. *Center for Disease Control and Prevention – National Center for Health Statistics.* Data Brief, Number 42, Sept 2010. Pg 1. <http://www.cdc.gov/nchs/data/databriefs/db42.pdf>

5   Opioid Painkiller Prescribing. *Center for Disease Control and Prevention – Vital Signs*, 2014. <http://www.cdc.gov/vitalsigns/opioid-prescribing/index.html>

6   Opioid Painkiller Prescribing: Where You Live Makes Difference. *Center for Disease Control and Prevention*, 2014. <http://www.cdc.gov/vitalsigns/pdf/2014-07-vitalsigns.pdf>

7   Manchikanti, L Singh, A. Therapeutic Opioids: A Ten-Year Perspective on the Complexities and Complications of the Escalating Use, Abuse, and Nonmedical Use of Opioids. *Journal of the American Society of Interventional Pain Physicians.* 11 (2S.), 2008. <http://www.painphysicianjournal.com/linkout_vw.php?issn=1533-3159&vol=11&page=S63>

8   Statement on Scientific Research on Prescription Drug Abuse to the U.S. Senate Subcommittee on Crime and Drugs, Judiciary Committee. *U.S. Department of Health & Human Services*, 2008. <http://www.hhs.gov/asl/testify/2008/03/t20080312a.html>

9   Ibid #2, Pg 20.

10   Goldberger, B, Thogmartin, J, Johnson, H, Paulozzi, L, Rudd, R, Ibrahimova, A. Drug Overdose Deaths – Florida, 2003-2009. *Center for Disease Control and Prevention – Morbidity and Mortality Weekly Report (MMWR)*, 2011. <http://www.cdc.gov/mmwr/preview/mmwrhtml/mm6026a1.htm>

11   Ibid #2, Pg 23.

12   Loya A, Stuart-Gonzalez, A, Rivera, J. Prevalence of Polypharmacy, Polyherbacy, Nutritional Supplement Use and Potential Product Interactions Among Older Adults Living on the United States-Mexico Border: A Descriptive, Questionnaire-based Study. *Drugs & Aging.* 26 (5): 423-436, 2009. <http://www.ncbi.nlm.nih.gov/pubmed/19552494>

13   Ibid #4.

14   Budnitz, D, Lovegrove, M, Shehab, N, Richards, C. Emergency Hospitalizations for Adverse Drug Events in Older Americans. *The New England Journal of Medicine.* 365 (2): 2002-2012, 2011. <http://www.nejm.org/doi/full/10.1056/NEJMsa1103053>

15   Lazarou, J, Pomeranz, B, Corey, P. Incidence of Adverse Drug Reactions in Hospitalized Patients: A Meta-Analysis of Prospective Studies. *The Journal of the American Medical Association.* 279 (15): 1200-1205, 1998. <http://jama.jamanetwork.com/article.aspx?articleid=187436>

Chapter Six

1   Starfield, B. Is US Health Really the Best in the World? *The Journal of the American Medical Association.* 284 (4): 483-485, 2010. <http://www.jhsph.edu/research/centers-and-institutes/johns-hopkins-primary-care-policy-center/Publications_PDFs/A154.pdf>

2   Ibid.

3   Zerehi, M. How Is a Shortage of Primary Care Physicians Affecting the Quality and Cost of Medical Care?: A Comprehensive Evidence Review. *American College of Physicians*, 2008. <http://www.acponline.org/advocacy/current_policy_papers/assets/primary_shortage.pdf>

4   Starfield, B, Shi, L, Macinko, J. Contribution of Primary Care to Health Systems and Health. *The Milbank Quarterly.* 83 (3): 457-502, 2005. <http://www.milbank.org/the-milbank-quarterly/search-archives/article/2089/contribution-of-primary-care-to-health-systems-and-health>

5   Ibid #3.

Chapter Seven

1   Tu, J, Pashos, C, Naylor, C, Chen, E, Normand, S, Newhouse, J, McNeil, B. Use of Cardiac Procedures and Outcomes in Elderly Patients with Myocadial Infarction in the United States and Canada. *The New England Journal of Medicine.* 336: 1500-1505, 1997. <http://www.nejm.org/doi/full/10.1056/NEJM199705223362106>

Chapter Eight

1   Kahn, J, Kronick, R, Kreger, M, Gans, D. The Cost of Health Insurance Administration in California: Estimates for Insurers, Physicians, and Hospitals. *Health Affairs.* 24 (6): 1629-1639, 2005. <http://content.healthaffairs.org/content/24/6/1629.full>

2   Woolhandler, S, Himmelstein, D. The Deteriorating Administrative Efficiency of the U.S. Health Care System. *The New England Journal of Medicine.* 324: 1253-1258, 1991. <http://www.nejm.org/doi/full/10.1056/NEJM199105023241805>

3   Woolhandler, S, Campbell, T, Himmelstein, D. Costs of Health Care Administration in the United States and Canada. *The New England Journal of Medicine.* 349: 768-775, 2003. <http://www.pnhp.org/publications/nejmadmin.pdf>

4   Pozen, A, Cutler, D. Medical Spending Differences in the United States and Canada: The Role of Prices, Procedures, and Administrative Expenses. *Inquiry Journal.* 47 (2): 124-134, 2010. <http://inq.sagepub.com/content/47/2/124.full.pdf+html>

5   Farrell, D, Jensen, E, Kocher, B, Lovegrove, N, Melhem, F, Mendonca, L, Parish, B. Accounting for the Cost of US Health Care: A New Look at Why Americans Spend More. *McKinsey Global Institute*, 2008. <http://www.mckinsey.com/insights/health_systems_and_services/accounting_for_the_cost_of_us_health_care>

6   Ungar, R. Busted: Health Insurers Secretly Spent Huge to Defeat Health Care Reform While Pretending to Support Obamacare. *Forbes*, 2012. <http://www.forbes.com/sites/rickungar/2012/06/25/ busted-health-insurers-secretly-spent-huge-to-defeat-health-care-reform-while-pretending-to-support-obamacare>

7   Cutler, D, Ly, D. The (Paper) Work of Medicine: Understanding International Medical Costs. *Journal of Economic Perspectives*. 25 (2): 3-25, 2011. <http://pubs.aeaweb.org/doi/pdfplus/10.1257/ jep.25.2.3>

8   New AMA Health Insurer Report Card Finds Increasing Inaccuracy in Claims Payment. *American Medical Association*, 2011. <http://www.ama-assn.org/ama/pub/news/news/ama-health-insurer-report-card.page>

Chapter Nine

1   Health at a Glance 2013: OECD Indicators. *Organisation for Economic Co-operation and Development*, 2013. <http://www. oecd-ilibrary.org/docserver/download/8113161e.pdf?expires=1421 768134&id=id&accname=guest&checksum=3F6F16F468BDB96 7 2A2A55A9FDDE6BC6>

2   Farrell, D, Jensen, E, Kocher, B, Lovegrove, N, Melhem, F, Mendonca, L, Parish, B. Accounting for the Cost of US Health Care: A New Look at Why Americans Spend More. *McKinsey Global Institute*, 2008. <http://www.mckinsey.com/insights/health_ systems_and_services/accounting_for_the_cost_of_us_health_ care>

3   Ibid.

4   Ibid.

5   Angell, M. Drug Companies & Doctors: A Story of Corruption. *The New York Review of Books*, 2009. <http://www.nybooks.com/ articles/archives/2009/jan/15/drug-companies-doctorsa-story-of-corruption>

6   Horton, R. Offline: What is Medicine's 4 Sigma? *The Lancet.* 385, 2015. <http://www.thelancet.com/pdfs/journals/lancet/PIIS0140-6736(15)60696-1.pdf>

Chapter Ten

1   Ali, T. Electronic Medical Record and Quality of Patient Care in the VA. *Medicine and Health/ Rhode Island, publication of the Rhode Island Medical Society.* 93 (1): 8-10, 2010. <https://www.rimed.org/medhealthri/2010-01/2010-01-8.pdf>

2   Evans, D, Nichol, W, Perlin, J. Effect of the Implementation of an Enterprise-Wide Electronic Health Record on Productivity in the Veterans Health Administration. *Health Economics, Policy and Law.* 1 (2): 163-169, 2006. <http://journals.cambridge.org/action/displayAbstract;jsessionid=7C274D08947B0625B3B540BEF2E70367.tomcat1?fromPage=online&aid=416400>

3   Jha, A, Perlin, J, Kizer, K, Dudley, R. Effect of the Transformation of the Veterans Affairs Health Care System on the Quality of Care. *The New England Journal of Medicine.* 348 (22): 2218-2227, 2003. <http://www.nejm.org/doi/full/10.1056/NEJMsa021899>

Chapter Eleven

1   Moriyama, I, Loy, R, Robb-Smith, A. History of the Statistical Classification of Diseases and Causes of Death. *Center for Disease Control and Prevention,* 2011. <http://www.cdc.gov/nchs/data/misc/classification_diseases2011.pdf>

2   ICD-9 to ICD-10: What and Why It's Being Implemented. *Experis.* <http://files.himss.org/HIMSSorg/Content/files/ICD9toICD10_Experis.pdf>

3   The Impact of Implementing ICD-10 on Physician Practices and Clinical Laboratories. *Nachimson Advisors, LLC*, 2008. <http://www.nachimsonadvisors.com/Documents/ICD-10%20Impacts%20 on%20Providers.pdf>

4   ICD-10 Cost Estimates Increased for Most Physicians. *American Medical Association News Room, 2014.* <http://www.ama-assn. org/ama/pub/news/news/2014/2014-02-12-icd10-cost-estimates-increased-for-most-physicians.page>

5   Medical Records and Health Information Technicians. *Bureau of Labor Statistics, 2014.* <http://www.bls.gov/ooh/healthcare/medical-records-and-health-information-technicians.htm>

6   A Survey of America's Physicians: Practice Patterns and Perspectives. *The Physicians Foundation, 2012.* <http://www.physiciansfoundation.org/uploads/default/Physicians_Foundation_2012_Biennial_Survey.pdf>

7   Ibid.

8   Deloitte 2013 Survey of U.S. Physicians. *Deloitte*, 2013. <http://www2.deloitte.com/content/dam/Deloitte/us/Documents/life-sciences-health-care/us-lshc-deloitte-2013-physician-survey-10012014.pdf>

9   IHS, Inc. The Complexities of Physician Supply and Demand: Projections from 2013 to 2025. *Association of American Medical Colleges*, 2015. Pg 32. <https://www.aamc.org/download/426242/data/ihsreportdownload.pdf>

10 Ibid.

Chapter Twelve

1   Ventola, C. Direct-to-Consumer Pharmaceutical Advertising: Therapeutic or Toxic? *Pharmacy and Therapeutics*. 36 (10): 669-684, 2011. <http://www.ncbi.nlm.nih.gov/pmc/articles/ PMC3278148>

2   Ibid.

3   Ibid.

4   Ibid.

5   Ibid.

6   Rubin, R. How Did Vioxx Debacle Happen? *USA Today*, 2004. <http://usatoday30.usatoday.com/news/health/2004-10-12-vioxx-cover_x.htm>

Chapter Thirteen

1   Starfield, B. Is U.S. Health Really the Best in the World? *The Journal of the American Medical Association*. 284 (4): 482-485, 2010. <http://www.jhsph.edu/research/centers-and-institutes/johns-hopkins-primary-care-policy-center/Publications_PDFs/A154.pdf>

2   Bunker, J. The Role of Medical Care in Contributing to Health Improvements within Societies. *International Journal of Epidemiology*. 30: 1260-1263, 2001. <http://ije.oxfordjournals.org/content/30/6/1260.full.pdf+html>

3   Kohn, L, Corrigan, J, Donaldson, M (eds). *To Err is Human: Building a Safer Health System*. Washington DC: National Academy Press, 2000. <http://books.nap.edu/openbook.php?record_id=9728&page=1>

Chapter Fourteen

1   Lazarou J, Pomeranz, B, Corey, P. Incidence of Adverse Drug Reactions in Hospitalized Patients: A Meta-Analysis of Prospective Studies. *The Journal of the American Medical Association*. 279 (15): 1200-1205, 1998. <http://jama.jamanetwork.com/article.aspx?articleid=187436>

2   Madeira, S, Melo, M, Porto, J, Monteiro, S, Pereira de Moura, J, Alexandrino, M, Alves Moura, J. The Disease We Cause: Iatrogenic Illness in a Department of Internal Medicine. *European Journal of Internal Medicine.* 18: 391-399, 2007. <http://rihuc.huc.min-saude.pt/bitstream/10400.4/1137/1/The%20diseases%20we%20cause.pdf>

3   Interim Update on 2013 Annual Hospital-Acquired Condition Rate and Estimates of Cost Savings and Deaths Averted From 2010 to 2013. *Agency for Healthcare Research and Quality*, 2013. <http://www.ahrq.gov/professionals/quality-patient-safety/pfp/interimhacrate2013.pdf>

4   Klevens, R, Edwards, J, Richards, C, Horan, T, Gaynes, R, Pollock, D, Cardo, D. Estimating Health Care-Associated Infections and Deaths in U.S. Hospitals, 2002. *Public Health Reports.* 122: 160-166, 2007. <http://www.publichealthreports.org/archives/issueopen.cfm?articleID=1813>

5   Ibid #2.

6   Bates, D, Spell, N, Cullen, D, Burdick, E, Laird, N, Petersen, L, Small, S, Sweitzer, B, Leape, L. The Costs of Adverse Drug Events in Hospitalized Patients. *The Journal of the American Medical Association.* 277 (4): 307-311, 1997. <http://jama.jamanetwork.com/article.aspx?articleid=413545>

7   Ibid #2.

8   Jarvis, W. Selected Aspects of the Socioeconomic Impact of Nosocomial Infections: Morbidity, Mortality, Cost, and Prevention. *Infection Control & Hospital Epidemiology.* 17 (8): 522-557, 2015. <http://journals.cambridge.org/action/displayAbstract?fromPage=o nline&aid=9309889&fileId=S019594170000480X>

9   Ibid #2.

10   Leape, L. Unnecessary Surgery. *Health Services Research.* 24 (3): 351-407, 1989. <http://www.ncbi.nlm.nih.gov/pmc/articles/PMC1065571/pdf/hsresearch00085-0066.pdf>

11   Ibid.

12   Eisler, P, Hansen, B. Doctors Perform Thousands of Unnecessary Surgeries. *USA Today*, 2013. <http://www.usatoday.com/story/news/nation/2013/06/18/unnecessary-surgery-usa-today-investigation/2435009>

13   Al-Khatib, S, Hellkamp, A, Curtis, J, Mark, D, Peterson, E, Sanders, F, Heidenreich, P, Hernandez, A, Curtis, L, Hammill, S. Non-Evidence-Based ICD Implantations in the United States: Results from the NCDR-ICD Registry. *The Journal of the American Medical Association*. 305 (1): 43-49, 2011.

<http://jama.jamanetwork.com/article.aspx?articleid=644551>

14   Epstein, N, Hood, D. Unnecessary Spinal Surgery: A Prospective 1-Year Study of One Surgeon's Experience. *Surgical Neurology International*. 2 (83), 2011. <http://www.surgicalneurologyint.com/article.asp?issn=2152-7806;year=2011;volume=2;issue=1;spage=83;epage=83;aulast=Epstein>

15   Sackett, D, Rosenburg, W, Gray, J, Haynes, J, Richardson, W. Evidence-based medicine: what it is and it isn't. *The British Medical Journal*. 312: 71–72, 1996. <http://www.ncbi.nlm.nih.gov/pubmed/8555924>

Chapter Fifteen

1   Kotlikoff, L. America's Hidden Credit Card Bill. *The New York Times*, 2014. <http://www.nytimes.com/2014/08/01/opinion/laurence-kotlikoff-on-fiscal-gap-accounting.html?_r=0>

2   The 2014 Long-Term Budget Outlook. *Congressional Budget Office*, 2014. <http://www.cbo.gov/publication/45471>

3   Reinhart, C, Rogoff, K. Growth in a Time of Debt. *National Bureau of Economic Research, Working Paper No. 15639*, 2010. <http://www.nber.org/papers/w15639.pdf>

Chapter Twenty

1 Mello, M. The Medical Liability Climate: The Calm Before Storms is the Time for Reforms. *Harvard Law School Petrie-Flom Center*, 2014. <http://blogs.law.harvard.edu/billofhealth/2014/10/31/the-medical-liability-climate-the-calm-between-storms-is-the-time-for-reforms>

2 10 Years of Tort Reform in Texas Bring Fewer Suits, Lower Payouts. *Insurance Journal*, 2013. <http://www.insurancejournal.com/news/southcentral/2013/09/03/303718.htm>

Chapter Twenty-Two

1 Oberlander, J. Unfinished Journey – A Century of Health Care Reform in the United States. *The New England Journal of Medicine*. 367: 585-590, 2012. <http://www.nejm.org/doi/full/10.1056/NEJMp1202111>

2 Timeline: History of Health Reform in the U.S. *The Henry J. Kaiser Family Foundation*, 2013. <http://kaiserfamilyfoundation.files.wordpress.com/2011/03/5-02-13-history-of-health-reform.pdf>

3 Palmer, K. A Brief History: Universal Health Care Efforts in the US. *Physicians for a National Health Program (PHNP)*, 1999. <http://www.pnhp.org/facts/a-brief-history-universal-health-care-efforts-in-the-us>

4 Ibid #1.
5 Ibid #2.
6 Ibid #2.
7 Ibid #1.
8 Ibid #3.
9 Ibid #2.
10 Ibid #2.
11 Ibid #2.
12 Ibid #1.

13   Hoffman, C. National Health Insurance – A Brief History of Reform Efforts in the U.S. *The Henry J. Kaiser Family Foundation – Focus on Health Reform*, 2009. <https://kaiserfamilyfoundation.files.wordpress.com/2013/01/7871.pdf>

14   Ibid #2.

15   Ibid #2.

16   Ibid #2.

17   Ibid #2.

18   Ibid #1.

19   Ibid #1.

20 Blumenthal, D, Abrams, M, Nuzum, R. The Affordable Care Act at 5 Years. *The New England Journal of Medicine.* 372: 2451-2458, 2015. <http://www.nejm.org/doi/full/10.1056/NEJMhpr1503614?af=R&rss=currentIssue>

21 Ibid #1.

22 Rubin, J. Obamacare Fallout. *The Washington Post*, 2013. <http://www.washingtonpost.com/blogs/right-turn/wp/2013/03/27/obamacare-fallout>

23 Accomplishments of the Affordable Care Act. *The Domestic Policy Council*, 2015. <https://www.whitehouse.gov/sites/default/files/docs/3-22-15_aca_anniversary_report.pdf>

24 Ibid #22.

25 Brill, S. Bitter Pill: Why Medical Bills Are Killing Us. *TIME*, 2013.   <http://time.com/198/bitter-pill-why-medical-bills-are-killing-us>

26   Key Facts about the Uninsured Population. *The Henry J. Kaiser Family Foundation – The Kaiser Commission on Medicaid and the Uninsured*, 2014.   <http://files.kff.org/attachment/key-facts-about-the-uninsured-population-fact-sheet>

Chapter Twenty-Three

1 The Long-Term Outlook for Health Care Spending. *Congressional Budget Office*, 2007. <http://www.cbo.gov/sites/default/files/11-13-lt-health.pdf>

2 Farrell, D, Jensen, E, Kocher, B, Lovegrove, N, Melhem, F, Mendonca, L, Parish, B. Accounting for the Cost of US Health Care: A New Look at Why Americans Spend More. *McKinsey Global Institute*, 2008. <http://www.mckinsey.com/insights/health_systems_and_services/accounting_for_the_cost_of_us_health_care>

3 Ibid #1.

4 Kotlikoff, L. U.S. is Bankrupt and We Don't Even Know It. *Bloomberg Business*, 2010. <http://www.bloomberg.com/news/articles/2010-08-11/u-s-is-bankrupt-and-we-don-t-even-know-commentary-by-laurence-kotlikoff>

5 Letter to Congress and President Obama. *The INFORM Act*. <http://www.theinformact.org/content/letter-congress-and-president-obama>

6 1000+ Economists, 15 Nobel Laureates, Endorse Bipartisan INFORM Act. *PR News Wire*, 2013. <http://www.prnewswire.com/news-releases/1000-economists-15-nobel-laureates-endorse-bipartisan-inform-act-228786001.html>

ABOUT THE AUTHOR

N.F. Hanna, M.D. has a total of almost 40 years of experience as a physician in both the United States and the United Kingdom. He has operated his own primary care practice in family and internal medicine in Jacksonville, Florida for the past 27 years. Dr. Hanna formerly served as associate editor of *Northeast Florida Medicine* for 10 years. He has written articles on a variety of topics, many of which are covered in this book.

Dr. Hanna was born and raised in Egypt, where he initially attended Assiut University College of Medicine in Upper Egypt and later continued on to graduate from Ain-Shams University College of Medicine in the capital city of Cairo in 1974. He then went on to receive post-graduate training in the U.K. He is a Licentiate of the Royal College of Physicians and a Member of the Royal College of Surgeons, London. He is a former college soccer player and award winner in poetry in his native language. Dr. Hanna and his wife Afaf live in Jacksonville, where they raised their three children: Amy, Amorette, and Andrew.

Made in the USA
Middletown, DE
27 May 2022